◆ 药学实验系列教材 ◆

药物化学实验

（中英双语）

Medicinal Chemistry Experiments

黄世亮　谭嘉恒　主编

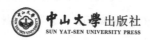
中山大学出版社
SUN YAT-SEN UNIVERSITY PRESS

·广州·

图书在版编目（CIP）数据

药物化学实验/黄世亮，谭嘉恒主编．—广州：中山大学出版社，2023.12
药学实验系列教材
ISBN 978 – 7 – 306 – 07957 – 2

Ⅰ.①药…　Ⅱ.①黄…②谭…　Ⅲ.①药物化学—化学实验—高等学校—教材
Ⅳ.①R914 – 33

中国国家版本馆 CIP 数据核字（2023）第 242695 号

YAOWU HUAXUE SHIYAN

出 版 人：王天琪
策划编辑：粟　丹　罗永梅
责任编辑：罗永梅
封面设计：曾　婷
责任校对：舒　思
责任技编：靳晓虹
出版发行：中山大学出版社
电　　话：编辑部 020 – 84110283，84113349，84111997，84110779，84110776
　　　　　　发行部 020 – 84111998，84111981，84111160
地　　址：广州市新港西路 135 号
邮　　编：510275　传　真：020 – 84036565
网　　址：http://www.zsup.com.cn　E-mail：zdcbs@mail.sysu.edu.cn
印　刷　者：广东虎彩云印刷有限公司
规　　格：787mm×1092mm　1/16　8 印张　205 千字
版次印次：2023 年 12 月第 1 版　2023 年 12 月第 1 次印刷
定　　价：28.00 元

本书编委会

黄世亮（中山大学药学院）

谭嘉恒（中山大学药学院）

曾优美（中山大学药学院）

前　言

　　药物化学实验是药学专业本科生学习的必修课。课程设立的主要目的是希望学生通过实验的方式深入了解药物化学的基本概念、实验技能和研究方法。同时，药物化学实验也会起到承上启下的作用，其先导基础课程为生物化学实验和有机化学实验。在综合学习了这些基础实验的单元操作后，可以为更高阶的实验（如药学综合大实验）打下基础。传统的药物化学实验教材大多强调合成与纯化过程，较少涉及化合物的活性及构效关系研究，而这部分往往是理论课的核心内容。这很容易造成实验课与理论课脱节的情况。但是，如果在药物化学实验课中加入化合物的设计、改造、活性测试及构效关系讨论等研究内容，则会导致实验课时和实验经费的大幅度增加，相关仪器设备也要进行相应的升级。针对这些问题，本教材在实验案例上进行了大量的优化，分别从课时、操作难易程度、仪器设备及试剂费用、安全性等方面进行比较与平衡。总的来说，本教材涉及以下几方面内容：

　　药物的合成和分离纯化。药物合成所涉及的反应类型主要有酯化反应、复分解反应、还原反应、氧化反应、重排反应及缩合反应等，合成中涉及的基本单元操作有萃取、滴加、干燥、蒸馏、重结晶、柱色谱法、薄层色谱法、无水操作、半微量操作等技术。

　　药物的理化性质分析。例如，熔点、红外光谱、核磁共振谱等，加强了产物的光谱学数据收集及结构的分析鉴定。

　　化合物的活性测定。学生将学习如何通过实验测定化合物的生物活性，包括化合物对酶的抑制活性等。这部分内容需要以生物化学实验为基础。

　　化合物构效关系的分析与总结。学生将通过实验了解化合物的不同衍生物结构对其生物活性、理化性质及给药方式的影响。除此之外，我们还强调学生需要综合利用现有的数据对实验过程和实验结果进行深入的讨论和分析。这不仅有助于提高学生发现问题和解决问题的能力，还可以帮助学生更好地理解药物化学相关理论知识，为今后从事药物研发等相关工作打下基础。

　　本教材的实验内容从性质上可以分为验证性实验、综合性实验和设计性实验。不同性质的实验难度有所不同。同时，本教材也是双语教材，学校可以根据学生的培养目标、培养方案、师资情况和实验室的具体条件进行选择。也可以将综合性实验进行模块拆分以适应不同学校的要求。

目 录
Contents

实验一 阿司匹林的合成（微波辅助合成）

一、实验目的

（1）了解微波辅助合成技术的原理。

（2）掌握酯化反应的原理，进一步练习固体有机物的分离、提纯操作。

（3）熟悉阿司匹林杂质检验的原理。

二、背景知识

微波是指波长为 1 mm 至 1 m、频率为 300 MHz 至 30 GHz 的电磁波，工业和民用的频率一般为 2.45 GHz。微波能量对材料有很强的穿透力，能对被照射物产生深层加热作用。对于微波加热促进有机反应的机理，目前较为普遍的看法是极性有机分子吸收微波辐射能量后每秒钟会产生几十亿次的偶极振动，产生热效应，使分子间的相互碰撞及能量交换次数增加，因而使有机反应速度加快。另外，电磁场对反应分子间行为的直接作用而引起的非热效应，也是微波促进有机反应的重要原因。与传统加热法相比，微波辅助合成反应速度可加快几倍至上千倍。目前，微波辅助合成已成为一项新兴的绿色有机合成技术。

阿司匹林（aspirin）是人们熟悉的解热镇痛非甾体抗炎药物，可由水杨酸和乙酸酐合成得到。其合成涉及水杨酸的乙酰化反应和固体有机物的分离提纯等基本操作。现行教材都采用酸催化法合成阿司匹林，这种方法存在反应时间相对较长、乙酸酐用量大和副产物多等缺点。本实验将微波辐射技术应用于阿司匹林的合成，并采用碱催化的方法，获得了很好的实验结果。和传统方法相比，该方法具有反应时间短（约为80 s）、产率高（92%）和物质消耗及污染少的特点。

三、实验原理

阿司匹林的合成如图 1-1 所示。

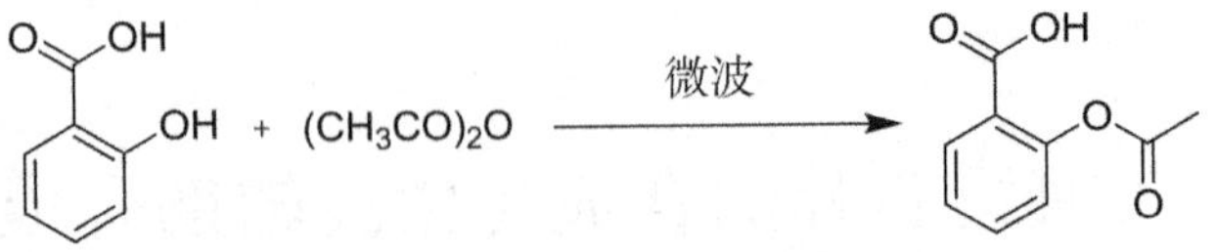

图1-1 阿司匹林的合成

四、实验方法

(一) 实验试剂

实验用试剂的规格、用量见表1-1。

表1-1 实验试剂规格和用量

试剂	规格	用量 （重量或体积）	物质的量/ mmol	摩尔比	安全信息
水杨酸	药用	1.0 g			
乙酸酐	分析纯	1.4 mL			
蒸馏水	—	适量			
乙醇	分析纯	10～15 mL			
Na$_2$CO$_3$	分析纯	0.1 g			
2% FeCl$_3$溶液	—	适量			

(二) 操作步骤

在50 mL干燥的圆底烧瓶中加入1.0 g（7.3 mmol）水杨酸和0.1 g Na$_2$CO$_3$，再用移液管加入1.4 mL（1.52 g，14.8 mmol）乙酸酐，轻轻摇匀，盖上瓶塞，在瓶塞与瓶子之间垫一张纸片，放入微波炉中，在390 W（中档）微波输出功率下，微波辐照60 s（或控制反应温度为80～90 ℃），拿出反应瓶，摇匀后，在同样功率下加热20 s。冷却至室温后，摩擦析晶，加入20 mL水，将混合物继续在冷水中冷却搅拌15 min，使之结晶完全。减压过滤，用少量冷水洗涤结晶2～3次，抽干，得阿司匹林粗产品。烘干，留样检测纯度和熔点。

每克粗产品用约10 mL的乙醇/水溶液（95%乙醇：水=1:2，v/v）重结晶（先加一半溶剂，回流不全溶，再加入剩下的一半），干燥，得白色晶状阿司匹林1.24 g（收率为92%，参考熔点为135～136 ℃）。产品的纯度可通过薄层色谱法（thin layer chromatography，TLC）的结果或对比纯品的熔点判断，其中的杂质还可用2% FeCl$_3$溶液检验，结构可以使用核磁共振法（nuclear magnetic resonance，NMR）和红外光谱法（infrared spectrometry，IR）进行鉴定。

五、附注

（1）乙酸酐应是新开瓶的。如果打开使用过且放置较长时间，使用时应重新蒸馏，收集 139～140 ℃的馏分。

（2）不同品牌的家用微波炉所用的微波条件略有不同，微波条件的选择以使反应温度达 80～90 ℃为原则。使用的微波功率一般为 350～500 W，微波辐照时间为 40～60 s，也可通过观察反应物是否完全溶解来判断。此外，微波炉不能长时间空载或近似空载操作，否则可能损坏磁控管。同一个微波炉可以同时进行多个反应，但要注意提前摸索反应时间和功率，以使反应完全。微波加热时，切勿将反应装置完全密闭，可在玻璃塞和瓶子间垫一纸片。

六、思考题

（1）微波加热的主要特点是什么？
（2）采用酸催化法合成阿司匹林，其主要副反应是什么？
（3）本实验中的碱除了选用 Na_2CO_3 外，还可以选用哪些物质？
（4）碱催化的优点是什么？
（5）在本实验中，微波功率为何选择 390 W 左右？
（6）为什么是水杨酸的羟基与乙酸酐反应，而不是羧基与乙酸酐反应？
（7）为什么选用乙醇/水溶液作为重结晶溶剂，而不选用乙酸乙酯？
（8）如何通过 NMR 和 IR 来鉴定阿司匹林？

Experiment 1　Synthesis of Aspirin (Microwave-Assisted Synthesis)

1　Learning Objectives

(1) To understand the principle of microwave-assisted synthesis technology.

(2) To master the principle of esterification reactions and further practice the separation and purification of solid organic matter.

(3) To familiarize the principles of testing aspirin impurities.

2　Introduction

Microwaves refer to electromagnetic waves with wavelengths of 1 mm – 1 m and frequencies of 300 MHz – 30 GHz. The frequency of industrial and civil microwaves is generally 2. 45 GHz. The microwave energy exhibits a high penetrating power on the material and can produce a deep heating effect on the irradiated material. Regarding the mechanism of promoting organic reactions through microwave heating, it is widely accepted that polar organic molecules generate billions of dipole vibrations per second when absorbing microwave energy. This generates thermal effects, increasing the number of intermolecular collisions and energy exchanges, accelerating the speed of organic reactions. In addition, the nonthermal effect caused by the direct effect of the electromagnetic field on the behavior of reaction molecules is also an important reason for promoting organic reactions by microwaves. Compared with the traditional heating method, the reaction speed of microwave heating can be several times to a thousand times faster. Recently, microwave-assisted synthesis has become a new green organic synthesis technology.

Aspirin is an antipyretic analgesic and nonsteroidal anti-inflammatory drug that can be synthesized from salicylic acid and acetic anhydride. Its synthesis involves basic reactions and operations such as acetylation of salicylic acid, separation, and purification of solid organic matter. The current synthesis methods usually involve acid catalysis to synthesize aspirin, which is disadvantaged by a relatively long reaction time, a large amount of acetic anhydride and many byproducts. In this experiment, microwave irradiation was applied to the synthesis of aspirin, the base catalysis method was applied, and good experimental results were obtained. Compared with the traditional method, the new method involves a short reaction time (about 80 s), high yield (92%) and less material consumption and pollution.

3　Experimental Principle

Synthesis of aspirin is shown in Figure 1 – 1.

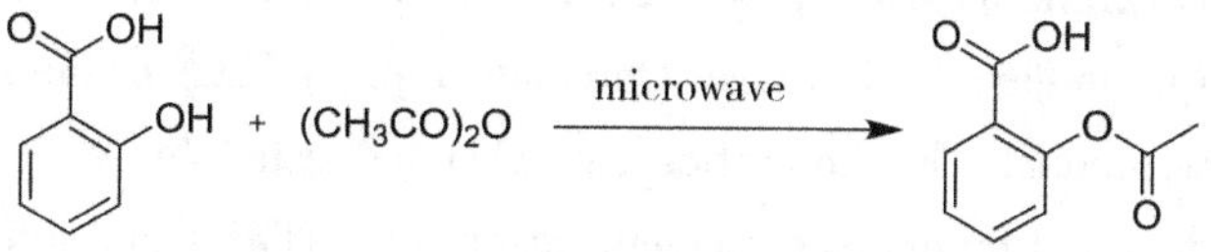

Figure 1 – 1 Synthesis of aspirin

4 Experimental Procedure

4. 1 Experimental Reagents

The experimental reagents are shown in Table 1 – 1.

Table 1 – 1 Dosage and specifications of experimental reagents

Reagents	Grade	Intended Amount	Amount of Substance/mmol	Molar Ratio	Safety Data
Salicylic acid	Medical grade	1. 0 g			
Acetic anhydride	Analytical pure	1. 4 mL			
Distilled water	—	Appropriate amount			
Ethanol	Analytical pure	10 – 15 mL			
Na_2CO_3	Analytical pure	0. 1 g			
2% $FeCl_3$ solution	—	Appropriate amount			

4. 2 Method

1. 0 g of salicylic acid (7. 3 mmol) and approximately 0. 1 g of Na_2CO_3 were added to a 50 mL dry round-bottom flask. Then, 1. 4 mL of acetic anhydride (1. 52 g, 14. 8 mmol) was added through a pipette and shaken gently. The flask stopper was covered, and a piece of paper was placed between the flask stopper and the flask. The sample was placed into a microwave oven and irradiated with a microwave output power of 390 W for 60 s (or control the reaction temperature of 80 – 90 ℃). The reaction flask was removed, shaken well, and heated at the same power for 20 s. After being cooled to room temperature, rub the flask wall to promote crystallization. Then, 20 mL of water was added, and the mixture was cooled and stirred in cold water for 15 min to complete crystallization. The solution was filtered under reduced pressure, and the residue was washed with a small amount of cold water 2 – 3 times to obtain aspirin, the crude product. The sample was dried and retained for the measurement of purity and melting point (m. p.).

Each gram of the crude product was recrystallized with approximately 10 mL of ethanol/ water solution (95% ethanol solution : water = 1 : 2, v/v) (half of the solvent was first added, if the product was not fully soluble, then the remaining half was added) and dried to obtain

1. 24 g of white crystalline aspirin (yield: 92%; reference m. p. : 135 – 136 ℃). The purity of the product can be judged by thin layer Chromatography (TLC) or the melting point of the comparatively pure product. The impurities can also be tested by 2% $FeCl_3$ solution. The structure can be identified by nuclear magnetic resonance (NMR) and infrared spectrometry.

5　Notes

(1) Acetic anhydride should be newly opened. If the solution has been opened and used for a long time, it should be redistilled and collected in 139 – 140 ℃ fractions.

(2) The microwave settings used by domestic microwave ovens of different brands may vary slightly. The conditions were selected based on the principle of reaching a reaction temperature of 80 – 90 ℃. Typically, a microwave power of 350 – 500 W was used, with a microwave irradiation time of 40 – 60 seconds, resulting in complete dissolution of the reactants. In addition, the microwave oven cannot be operated for a long time without a load or nearly without a load; otherwise, the magnetron may be damaged. Multiple reactions can be placed in the same microwave oven at the same time, but it is necessary to explore the reaction time and power in advance to complete the reaction. When microwave heating was performed, do not seal the reaction device completely. A piece of paper can be placed between the glass stopper and the flask.

6　Questions

(1) What are the main characteristics of microwave heating?

(2) If aspirin is synthesized by acid catalysis, what are the main side reactions?

(3) In addition to using Na_2CO_3 as an alkali, what other substances can be used as an alkali?

(4) What are the advantages of alkali catalysis?

(5) In the experiment, why is the microwave power set at approximately 390 W?

(6) Why does the hydroxyl group of salicylic acid, instead of the carboxyl group, react with acetic anhydride?

(7) Why is ethanol/water solution used as the recrystallization solvent instead of ethyl acetate?

(8) How is aspirin identified by NMR and infrared spectrum?

实验二 葡萄糖酸锌的合成

一、实验目的

(1) 掌握离子交换树脂分离纯化的原理、方法与操作。
(2) 了解当前合成葡萄糖酸锌的各种方法。
(3) 掌握通过多步化学反应合成药物的思路和策略。

二、背景知识

葡萄糖酸锌（zinc gluconate）分子式为 $C_{12}H_{22}O_{14}Zn$，分子量为 455.68，一般以无水物或含 3 个分子结合水（分子量为 509.73）的形式存在。本品为白色粗粉或结晶性粉末，易溶于水，极难溶于乙醇。葡萄糖酸锌为有机补锌剂，对比无机补锌剂，其对胃部刺激小，更易被吸收，被广泛应用于保健品和药品中，对锌缺乏症患者有重要的作用。

三、实验原理

葡萄糖酸锌的合成如图 2-1 所示。

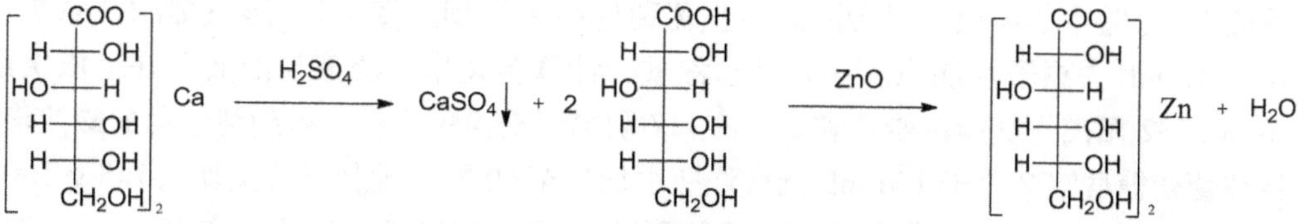

图 2-1 葡萄糖酸锌的合成

四、实验方法

(一) 实验试剂

实验用试剂的规格和用量见表 2-1。

表 2-1　实验试剂规格和用量

试剂	规格	用量 (重量或体积)	物质的量/ mmol	摩尔比	安全信息
8% H_2SO_4 溶液	—	31 mL (2.3 g 98%浓 H_2SO_4 溶液， 30 mL 水)			
葡萄糖酸钙	药用	10 g			
ZnO	分析纯	1.8 g			
732 阳离子交换树脂	—	约 20 mL (浸泡后体积)			
717 阴离子交换树脂	—	约 20 mL (浸泡后体积)			
2 mol/L HCl 溶液	—	约 100 mL			
1 mol/L NaOH 溶液	—	约 100 mL			
无水乙醇	分析纯	适量			
活性炭	—	适量			

(二) 操作步骤

在 100 mL 三颈烧瓶中加入 31 mL 8% H_2SO_4 溶液于 90 ℃ 水浴加热，称取 10 g 葡萄糖酸钙，在磁力搅拌下，分次向 H_2SO_4 溶液中加入葡萄糖酸钙粉，30 min 加完，反应 1 h (搅拌尽量快，但要注意防止葡萄糖酸钙溅到瓶壁上)。趁热抽滤，滤饼用 10～15 mL 去离子水洗涤。滤饼烘干称重，计算转化率。滤液与洗液合并，依次经 20 mL 732 阳离子交换树脂柱和 20 mL 717 阴离子交换树脂柱，得到纯葡萄糖酸溶液。将纯葡萄糖酸溶液置于 100 mL 圆底烧瓶中加热至 60 ℃，搅拌下分批加入 1.8 g ZnO，加完后 pH = 5～6。如果颜色过深，可同时加入活性炭脱色，搅拌反应 40 min，趁热抽滤得澄清溶液，滤饼烘干称重，计算实际消耗氧化锌的量。滤液加热减压蒸除多余的水分至 20 mL 左右，冷却后加入 10 mL 无水乙醇，冰水浴下不断摩擦器壁析出结晶。抽滤，先用少量预冷过的 50% 乙醇溶液洗涤，再用较大量无水乙醇洗涤，干燥脱水得白色粗产品，每克粗产品用 3～4 mL 水重结晶 (加热完全溶解粗产品后加入一半量的无水乙醇)。测产品的熔点，注意观察熔点管内样品性状的变化。

五、附注

（1）不管是阳离子交换柱还是阴离子交换柱，拿到柱子后，首先清洗干净，擦干塞子后涂凡士林，然后用水试漏，证明柱子是密封的才可以使用。阳离子交换树脂预先用 2 mol/L HCl 溶液、阴离子交换树脂预先用 1 mol/L NaOH 溶液浸泡过夜备用。

（2）732 阳离子交换树脂柱的处理方法：树脂用去离子水上柱后，用 50 mL 去离子水洗涤，再用 100 mL 2 mol/L HCl 溶液洗涤，流速为 5 ～ 10 mL/min，最后再用去离子水洗涤至流出液 pH = 6 ～ 7。将液面流至与树脂面相平，备用。

（3）717 阴离子交换树脂柱的处理方法：树脂用去离子水上柱后，用 50 mL 去离子水洗涤，再用 100 mL 1 mol/L NaOH 溶液洗涤，流速为 5 ～ 10 mL/min，最后用去离子水洗涤至 pH = 7 ～ 8。将液面流至与树脂面相平，备用。

（4）阳离子交换树脂柱（上）和阴离子交换树脂柱（下）串联使用。上样后，继续使用去离子水进行洗涤。整个过程不断检测阴离子交换树脂柱流出洗脱液 pH 的变化，收集所有 pH < 4 的样品。洗脱液 pH > 4 时停止接收。

（5）若阴、阳离子交换不完全，最后所得的产品难以析出结晶，得到黏稠状液体。

（6）氧化锌颗粒很细，易透过滤纸，需要在同一张滤纸上重复抽滤多次直至液体澄清为止。

（7）若采用电热套加热，容易局部过热，使产品焦化变色。若剩余水太少，析出的固体发黏，且包含大量杂质，不利于抽滤和洗涤；若剩余水太多，产品析出量少，产率降低。

（8）产品纯度越高，越易析出固体，可以加入晶种以促进固体析出。若时间允许，可以不摩擦，静置过夜，析出产品的质量和纯度都会有所提高。加入乙醇过多会使杂质也析出，产品有可能呈树脂状。若析出困难，可加入大量乙醇，析出树脂状物质，倒去上清液，重复上述操作两次进行重结晶，可得到合格的产品。

六、思考题

（1）查阅文献，综述目前葡萄糖酸锌的制备方法，比较不同方法之间的优缺点。

（2）葡萄糖酸钙与 H_2SO_4 反应后溶液经 732 阳离子交换树脂柱和 717 阴离子交换树脂柱的目的是什么？

（3）反应后的溶液能否先经阴离子交换树脂柱处理再经阳离子交换树脂柱处理？说明原因。

（4）通过得到的 $CaSO_4$ 的量、收集的洗脱液的体积、反应中 ZnO 的消耗量、粗品及精品的产量这些数据，分析实验可能出现的问题，对本次实验进行总结。

（5）析出固体，抽滤后，为什么先用少量预冷的 50% 乙醇溶液洗涤，再用大量的无水乙醇洗涤？

　　（6）从阴离子交换树脂柱流出的洗脱液应该是酸性的还是碱性的？分析原因。

　　（7）查阅文献，对最后产品熔点测定过程中出现的现象进行分析和解释。

Experiment 2   Synthesis of Zinc Gluconate

1   Learning Objectives

(1) To master the principle, method and operation of separation and purification of ion exchange resin.

(2) To understand the current various methods of synthesizing zinc gluconate.

(3) To master the ideas and strategies of synthesizing drugs through multistep chemical reactions.

2   Introduction

The molecular formula of zinc gluconate is $C_{12}H_{22}O_{14}Zn$, with a molecular weight of 455.68. Zinc gluconate is usually anhydrous or contains 3 molecules of crystalliferous water (molecular weight: 509.73) and is white powder or crystalline powder. The powder is easily soluble in water and extremely insoluble in ethanol. Zinc gluconate is an organic zinc fortifier. Compared with inorganic zinc supplements, zinc gluconate causes less irritation to the stomach and is easier to be absorbed. It is widely used in health care products and drugs and plays an important role for patients with zinc deficiency.

3   Experimental Principle

Synthesis of zinc gluconate is shown in Figure 2 – 1.

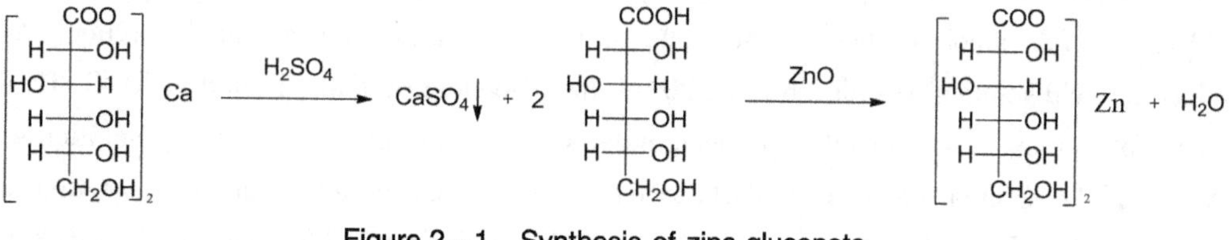

Figure 2 – 1   Synthesis of zinc gluconate

4   Experimental Procedure

4.1   Experimental Reagents

The experimental reagents are shown in Table 2 – 1.

Table 2 – 1   Dosage and specifications of experimental reagents

Reagents	Grade	Intended Amount	Amount of Substance/mmol	Molar Ratio	Safety Data
8% H_2SO_4 solution	—	31 mL (2.3 g 98% H_2SO_4 solution and 30 mL water)			

Table 2 − 1（Continued）

Reagents	Grade	Intended Amount	Amount of Substance/mmol	Molar Ratio	Safety Data
Calcium gluconate	Medical grade	10 g			
ZnO	Analytical pure	1.8 g			
732 cation exchange resin	—	15 − 20 mL			
717 anion exchange resin	—	15 − 20 mL			
2 mol/L HCl solution	—	About 100 mL			
1 mol/L NaOH solution	—	About 100 mL			
Anhydrous ethanol	Analytical pure	Appropriate amount			
Activated carbon	—	Appropriate amount			

4.2　Method

31 mL of 8% H_2SO_4 solution was added to a 100 mL three-neck flask and heated in a 90 ℃ water bath. 10 g of calcium gluconate was added in portions under magnetic stirring for 30 min and was reacted for 1 h（Stir as fast as possible, but be careful not to splash the calcium gluconate on the wall of the flask）. The liquid was hot filtered, and the filter cake was washed with 10 − 15 mL of deionized water. The filter cake was dried and weighed, and the conversion rate of calcium gluconate was calculated. The filtrate was combined with the washing solution and then passed through a 20 mL of 732 cation exchange resin column and a 20 mL of 717 anion exchange resin column to obtain pure gluconic acid solution. Pure gluconic acid solution was placed in a 100 mL round-bottom flask and heated to 60 ℃. Then, 1.8 g of zinc oxide was added in portions under stirring. After that, the pH of the solution was 5 − 6. If the solution color is too dark, activated carbon can be added at the same time for decolorization. Then, the mixture was stirred for 40 min, and a hot filter was conducted. Filter cake was dried and weighed, and the actual consumption of zinc oxide was calculated. The filtrate was heated and evaporated under reduced pressure to remove excess water to approximately 20 mL. After cooling, 10 mL of ethanol was added, and crystal was continuously precipitated by rubbing the wall of the container in an ice water bath. After filtration, the filter cake was washed with a small amount of 50% precooled ethanol and then a large amount of anhydrous ethanol and dried to obtain a white crude product. Each gram of crude product was recrystallized with 3 − 4 mL of water（heated to dissolve all the crude product, then adding half the amount of ethanol）. The melting point was measured, and the sample changes in the melting point tube were observed.

5　Notes

（1）After obtaining the column, clean it, wipe the stopper dry and apply vaseline, and then test for leaks with water to ensure the column is sealed before use. The cation exchange resin was presoaked in 2 mol/L HCl solution, and the anion exchange resin was presoaked in 1 mol/L NaOH solution overnight.

(2) Method of processing the 732 cation exchange resin column: The resin was washed with 50 mL of deionized water, then washed with 100 mL of 2 mol/L HCl solution at a flow rate of 5 – 10 mL/min, and finally washed with deionized water until the effluent pH was 6 – 7. The liquid surface was flowed to the resin surface.

(3) Method of processing the 717 anion exchange resin column: The resin was washed with 50 mL of deionized water, then washed with 100 mL of 1 mol/L NaOH solution at a flow rate of 5 – 10 mL/min, and finally washed with deionized water until the effluent pH was 7 – 8. The liquid surface was flowed to the resin surface.

(4) Cation exchange resin column (upper) and anion exchange resin column (lower) were used in series. After the sample was loaded, the sample was eluted using deionized water. The pH of the anion resin eluent was continuously detected, and collect all eluent with pH < 4. The collection of eluent was stopped when pH > 4.

(5) If the exchange of anions and cations is incomplete, the final product is difficult to precipitate and is viscous liquid.

(6) Zinc oxide particles are very fine and easily pass through filter paper. It is necessary to repeat the same process with filter paper several times until the liquid is clear.

(7) If heated with an electric heating jacket, it is easy for local overheating and product coking discoloration to occur. If too little residual water is left, the precipitated solid will be sticky and contain many impurities, making it difficult to filter and wash. If too much residual water is left, the product yield will be low and the overall yield will decrease.

(8) The higher the purity of the product, the easier the solid precipitates. Adding some seed crystals can promote solid precipitation. If time allows, leaving the crude product overnight without shaking and friction can improve the quality and purity of the precipitated product. Excessively adding ethanol will also precipitate impurities, and the product may be resin-like. However, if the product is difficult to precipitate, a large amount of ethanol can be added. In this method, the resin-like substance is precipitated, the supernatant is discarded, the same operation is repeated twice for the recrystallization; then, the qualified products are obtained.

6 Questions

(1) Review the current methods of preparing zinc gluconate and compare the advantages and disadvantages of different methods.

(2) What is the purpose of eluting the solution through 732 cation exchange resin column and 717 anion exchange resin column after calcium gluconate reacts with H_2SO_4?

(3) Can the reaction solution be treated with an anion exchange resin column before a

cation exchange resin column? Explain the reason.

(4) Analyze the problems that may occur in the experiment and summarize this experiment through the amount of the obtained $CaSO_4$, the volume of the eluent collected by the column chromatography, the consumption of zinc oxide in the reaction, and the yield of crude products and pure products.

(5) Why is the sample washed with a small amount of 50% ice ethanol and then washed with a large amount of anhydrous ethanol after the precipitate is filtered?

(6) Should the eluent from anion exchange resin have an acidic or basic pH, Why?

(7) Analyze and explain the phenomenon that occurs when measuring the melting point of the final product by consulting the literature.

实验三　沙利度胺的合成

一、实验目的

（1）了解沙利度胺的发展历史及其对药物研发的意义。

（2）熟练掌握 TLC 监测反应过程。

（3）掌握酸酐与胺的缩合反应机理。

二、背景知识

沙利度胺（thalidomide）（图 3 - 1）又名反应停，是一种谷氨酸衍生物，该药于 20 世纪 50 年代首先在西德上市，有镇静和止吐的作用，由于疗效显著且无严重不良反应，临床上被广泛用于治疗妊娠恶心和呕吐等症状。但在该药应用的几年内，世界上却发生了数万例罕见的儿童海豹肢畸形病例，在确认是由服用反应停引起之后，该药物在 20 世纪 60 年代初即被禁用。当时，美国食品药品监督管理局（Food and Drug Administration，FDA）以该药为孕妇用药却没有提供对胎儿影响的数据为由，未批准该药品在美国上市，从而避免了这种药物给美国带来的伤害。这一事件促使 FDA 推出新的药品审批法案，要求必须证明药品的有效性和安全性后，方可上市销售。该法案可以说是现代药品监管的里程碑式法案，对全球新药审评体系的发展产生了深远的影响。"反应停"事件也是现代药物研发中最常被引用的经典案例。

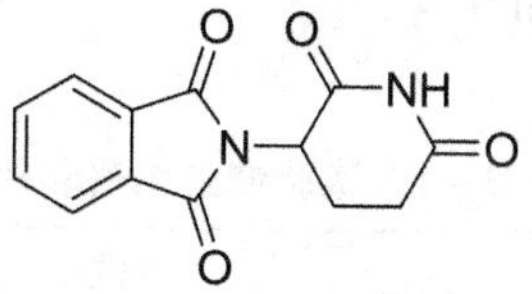

图 3 - 1　沙利度胺

近年来，有研究发现，沙利度胺具有抗炎、免疫调节、抗新生血管生成、抑制肿瘤坏死因子 - α（tumor necrosis factor-α，TNF-α）的生成等多种药理作用。因此，沙利度胺再次被广泛应用于多种严重疾病的治疗，2006 年，其被 FDA 正式批准用于治疗多发性骨髓瘤。沙利度胺的两种旋光异构体具有不同的作用。其中，R（ + ）起镇静催眠作用，S（ - ）则与不良反应致畸和免疫抑制作用有关。由于沙利度胺的单旋体在人体正常的代谢中会自动生成消旋体，因此不能通过单旋体给药消除不良反应。

结构的改造可以减少沙利度胺的副作用，由此发现的泊马度胺（pomalidomide）（图3-2）和来那度胺（lenalidomide）（图3-3）目前已成为抗肿瘤药物的"明星"分子。来那度胺的销售额在2020年位居全球药物（包含生物药、化药和疫苗）销售额第4位，高达140亿美元。另外，沙利度胺及其衍生物可以特异性结合羟脑苷脂（Cereblon，CRBN）蛋白，而CRBN在蛋白泛素化降解过程中起着重要作用。尽管沙利度胺类药物致畸的作用也是由结合CRBN后促进了转录因子人类婆罗双树样基因4（spalt-like transcription factor 4，SALL4）的降解而引起的，但基于此原理而开发的PROTAC蛋白降解技术，很有可能引领下一阶段抗肿瘤药物的研发风潮。

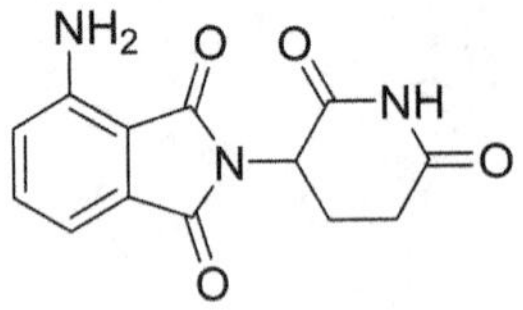

图3-2 泊马度胺

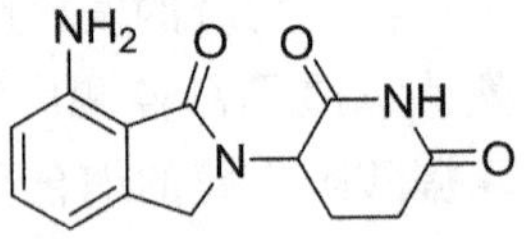

图3-3 来那度胺

三、实验原理

沙利度胺的合成如图3-4所示。

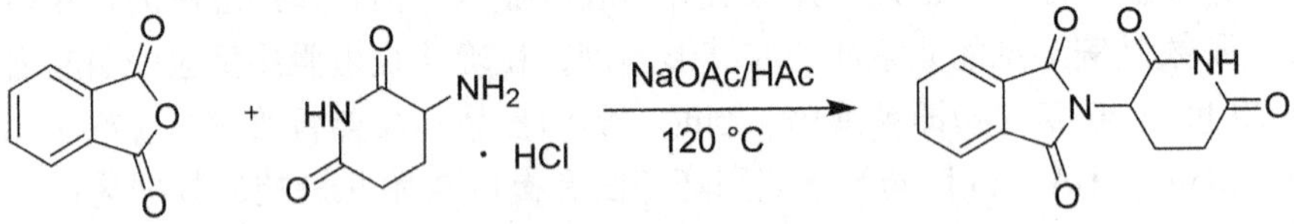

图3-4 沙利度胺的合成

四、实验方法

（一）实验试剂
实验用试剂的规格和用量见表3-1。

表3-1 实验试剂规格和用量

试剂	规格	用量（重量或体积）	物质的量/mmol	摩尔比	安全信息
邻苯二甲酸酐	分析纯	1 g			
3-氨基-2，6-哌啶二酮盐酸盐	分析纯	1.2 g			
乙酸钠	分析纯	1.5 g			
乙酸	分析纯	10 mL			

（二）操作步骤

取 1 g 邻苯二甲酸酐，1.2 g 3 - 氨基 - 2，6 - 哌啶二酮盐酸盐及 1.5 g 乙酸钠溶于 10 mL 乙酸中，120 ℃搅拌 1.5 h，TLC 监测反应过程。在确认反应结束后，冷却至室温，加入 25 mL 冷水稀释，0 ℃搅拌 30 min，抽滤，烘干得到灰色固体。测定产品的熔点（参考熔点为 269～271 ℃），并通过 ^{1}H-NMR、TLC 检测纯度，计算产率。

五、思考题

（1）在反应中，乙酸钠和乙酸的作用是什么？还可以用什么来代替？

（2）请问是否可以采用与沙利度胺类似的原料和方法合成泊马度胺？请画出泊马度胺的合成路线。

（3）根据沙利度胺、泊马度胺和来那度胺的结构特点，初步估计该类化合物的结构保守区域，以及 3 个环中哪个环对活性影响最大？

（4）为什么反应后可以采用冷水稀释、抽滤洗涤的方法得到产品？

Experiment 3　Synthesis of Thalidomide

1　Learning Objectives

(1) To understand the developmental history of thalidomide and its significance for drug research and development.

(2) To master TLC to detect the reaction process.

(3) To master the condensation reaction mechanism of anhydride with amine.

2　Introduction

Thalidomide (Figure 3 – 1) is glutamate derivative. This drug was first marketed in West Germany in the 1950s. It has sedative and antiemetic effects, and is mainly used to treat pregnancy nausea, vomiting and other symptoms. Because of its remarkable curative effect, mild nature and few adverse reactions, thalidomide has been widely used worldwide. However, within a few years of application of the drug, tens of thousands of cases of children with phocomelia, which were extremely rare in the past, have occurred worldwide and were confirmed to be caused by thalidomide. Therefore, the drug was banned in the early 1960s. Because the FDA noticed the potential harm of the drug, the drug was not approved for the market in the United States, thus citizens in the United States were not harmed by the drug. At the same time, this event prompted the FDA to introduce a new drug approval law, which requires that the effectiveness and safety of a drug be proven before it can be marketed and sold. The law is a milestone in modern drug regulation, and has had a profound impact on the development of global new drug evaluation systems. The "thalidomide tragedy" is also one of the most commonly cited classic cases in modern drug development.

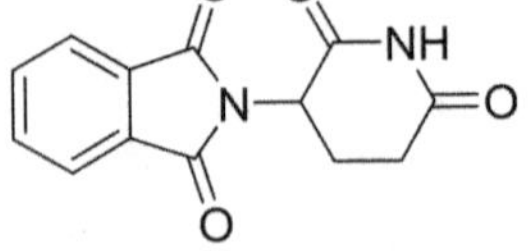

Figure 3 – 1　Thalidomide

In recent years, it has been found that thalidomide exhibits anti-inflammatory, immunomodulatory and antiangiogenic effects and can inhibit tumor necrosis factor-α (TNF-α). The drug has been widely used again in the treatment of many serious diseases and symptoms. In 2006, thalidomide was officially approved by the FDA for the treatment of multiple myeloma. The essence of thalidomide's pharmacological action and adverse reaction originates from its two optical isomers. $R(+)$ plays a sedative and hypnotic role, while $S(-)$ plays a teratogenic and immunosuppressive role. Because thalidomide can automatically generate racemates under physiological conditions and metabolism *in vivo*, racemates are also used clinically.

In order to reduce the side effects of thalidomide, pomalidomide (Figure 3 − 2) and lenalidomide (Figure 3 − 3) were discovered through structural modification. Currently, these two drugs have become star molecules in the field of anticancer drugs. Lenalidomide ranked fourth in the global sales of drugs (including biological drugs, chemical drugs and vaccines) in 2020, reaching 14 billion dollars. Moreover, thalidomide and its derivatives can specifically bind the Cereblon (CRBN) protein, and CRBN plays an important role in the process of protein ubiquitination and degradation. The teratogenic effect of thalidomide drugs is caused by the degradation of the spalt-like transcription factor 4 (SALL4) after it binds CRBN. However, the protein degradation technology of PROTAC developed based on this principle will likely provide a trend in antitumor drug research and development in the next stage.

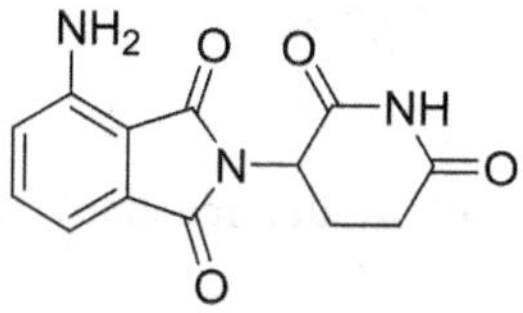

Figure 3 − 2　Pomalidomide 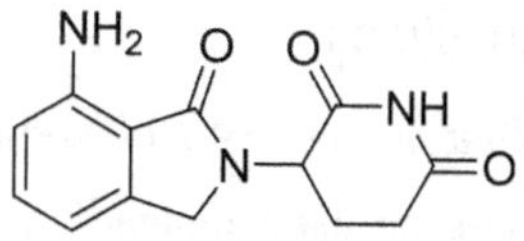　　　　Figure 3 − 3　Lenalidomide

3　Experimental Principle

Synthesis of thalidomide is shown in Figure 3 − 4.

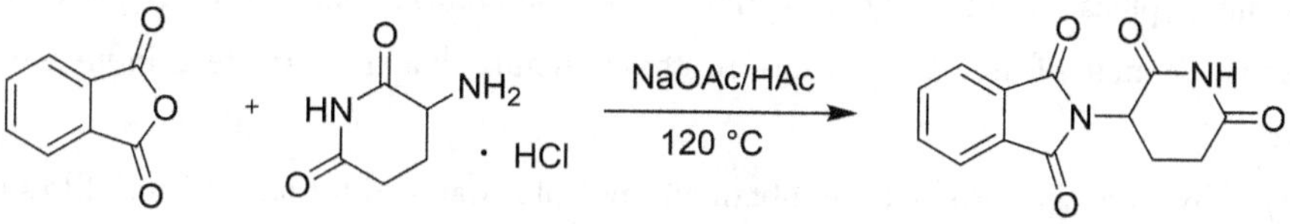

Figure 3 − 4　Synthesis of thalidomide

4　Experimental Procedure

4.1　Experimental Reagents

The experimental reagents are shown in Table 3 − 1.

Table 3 − 1　Dosage and specifications of experimental reagents

Reagents	Grade	Intended Amount	Amount of Substance/mmol	Molar Ratio	Safety Data
Phthalic anhydride	Analytical pure	1 g			

Table 3 − 1(Continued)

Reagents	Grade	Intended Amount	Amount of Substance/mmol	Molar Ratio	Safety Data
3-Amino-2, 6-piperidinedione hydrochloride	Analytical pure	1. 2 g			
Sodium acetate	Analytical pure	1. 5 g			
Acetic acid	Analytical pure	10 mL			

4. 2   Method

1 g of phthalic anhydride, 1. 2 g of 3-amino-2, 6-piperidinedione hydrochloride, and 1. 5 g of sodium acetate were dissolved in 10 mL of acetic acid and stirred at 120 ℃ for 1. 5 h, with the whole reaction process monitored by TLC. After confirming that the reaction was complete, cool to room temperature; then, 25 mL of cold water was added for dilution and the solution was stirred at 0 ℃ for 30 min, filtered by suction, and dried to obtain gray solid. The melting point (reference m. p. : 269 − 271 ℃) of the product was measured, the purity was detected by ^{1}H-NMR and TLC, and the yield was calculated.

5   Questions

(1) What is the role of sodium acetate and acetic acid in the reaction? What other conditions can be used instead?

(2) Is it possible to synthesize pomalidomide using materials and methods similar to thalidomide? Please draw the synthetic route of pomalidomide.

(3) According to the structural characteristics of thalidomide, pomalidomide and lenalidomide, please preliminarily estimate the structural conserved regions of these compounds. Which of the three rings in the structure has the greatest influence on the activity?

(4) Why can the product be obtained by cold water dilution, suction filtration and washing after the reaction?

实验四　盐酸二甲双胍的合成

一、实验目的

（1）了解盐酸二甲双胍的药学意义。

（2）了解现有合成盐酸二甲双胍的方法。

（3）掌握无溶剂法合成盐酸二甲双胍的优缺点。

二、背景知识

糖尿病的患病率和发病率在世界范围内不断增加，并且，糖尿病患者还有可能同时患上心血管疾病，而心血管疾病是全世界糖尿病患者最重要的并发症及主要死因。近60%的糖尿病患者死于心血管疾病。

二甲双胍（metformin）是双胍类口服降血糖药物，是目前全球治疗2型糖尿病的一线药物。二甲双胍于20世纪50年代在欧洲上市，但直到1994年12月30日才得到美国FDA的批准。与磺脲类药物不同，二甲双胍对胰岛素的分泌无影响，也不刺激胰岛β细胞，因此对正常人的血糖无影响。二甲双胍抗高血糖的作用机制包括减少肠道对葡萄糖的吸收，增加从血液到组织中的葡萄糖摄取，减少肝脏中的葡萄糖生成，减少葡萄糖利用对胰岛素的需求。近年来的研究发现，二甲双胍具有多种药理作用，如改善血脂、调节肠道菌群和人体免疫、预防和治疗多种肿瘤，在动物水平甚至显示具有预防衰老和延长寿命的作用。二甲双胍新的药理作用仍然在不断发现和挖掘中。

二甲双胍盐酸盐的合成方法主要通过盐酸二甲胺与二氰二胺的亲核加成反应得到。从反应条件上可分为溶剂法和无溶剂法，溶剂法是工业合成的主要方法，由于二氰二胺中氰基碳的正电性较弱，因此，一般采用高沸点溶剂作介质，如二甲苯、二苯醚等，也可采用水作为溶剂，在高压密闭反应体系中进行反应。

三、实验原理

本实验采用无溶剂反应体系，反应式如图4－1所示。

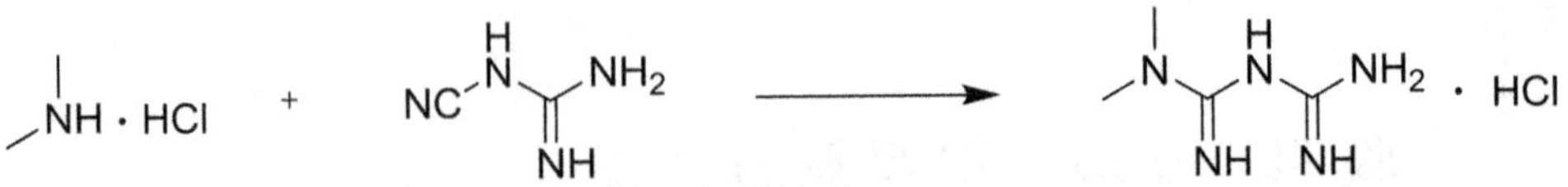

图 4 - 1   盐酸二甲双胍的合成

四、实验方法

(一) 实验试剂

实验用试剂的规格和用量见表 4 - 1。

表 4 - 1   实验试剂规格和用量

试剂	规格	用量 （重量或体积）	物质的量/ mmol	摩尔比	安全信息
盐酸二甲胺	分析纯	2.45 g			
二氰二胺	分析纯	2.49 g			
95%乙醇	分析纯	每克粗品约 20 mL			

(二) 操作步骤

在三口烧瓶中加入 2.45 g 盐酸二甲胺和 2.49 g 二氰二胺。插入温度计，并装上干燥管，搅拌加热升温至 140 ℃使物料呈熔融状态，加热搅拌至反应物凝固，继续反应 1 h，停止反应。每克粗产物用大约 20 mL 95%乙醇进行重结晶，放置后析出大量白色针状晶体。抽滤，结晶物用 95%乙醇洗涤，洗涤后的产物在红外快速干燥箱中烘干，称重，计算收率，测量熔点、IR 和 ^{1}H-NMR。（参考收率为 40%～60%，精品熔点为 220～225 ℃）

五、附注

(1) 采用无溶剂法合成盐酸二甲双胍时，随着反应温度的升高，烧瓶中的混合物从熔融状态到重新凝结为固体所需时间逐渐缩短。例如，100 ℃下大约需要 100 min，120 ℃下大约需要 45 min，而 140 ℃下大约需要 35 min。但是，需要注意的是，当温度超过 180 ℃时，有可能不再凝结为固体，通过产物间及产物与原料间的反应，有可能生成一系列三聚氰胺类衍生物（图 4 - 2），使产物收率和质量大幅度降低。因此，该反应的关键是温度的控制。

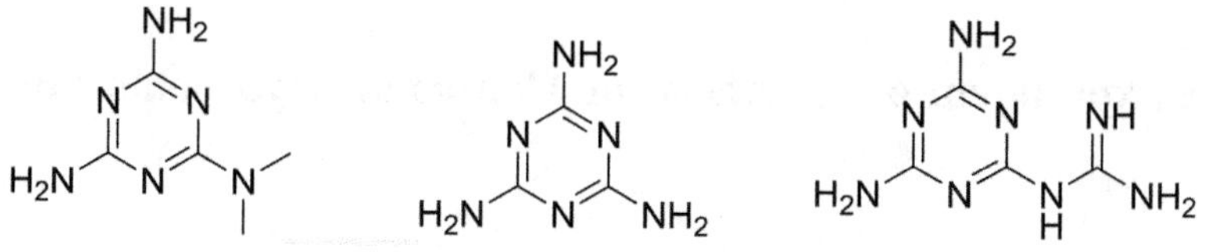

图4-2　三聚氰胺类衍生物

（2）重结晶的时候，乙醇含水量对二甲双胍的溶解度有巨大的影响。例如，采用80%乙醇重结晶时，每克粗品只需要5～6 mL的溶剂，而采用无水乙醇重结晶时，则需要大约40 mL的溶剂。

六、思考题

（1）查阅文献，比较溶剂法和无溶剂法合成盐酸二甲双胍的优缺点。

（2）请探讨合成二甲双胍的反应中三聚氰胺类杂质生成的机理。

（3）如果采用溶剂法进行反应，苯、甲苯和二甲苯哪种溶剂比较合适？理由是什么？

（4）为何反应物先熔融，继续反应后再凝固？

（5）对于IR和^{1}H-NMR图谱，哪个图谱更容易鉴别是否有原料二氰二胺的残留？

Experiment 4   Synthesis of Metformin Hydrochloride

1   Learning Objectives

(1) To understand the pharmaceutical significance of metformin hydrochloride.

(2) To understand the existing methods of synthesizing metformin hydrochloride.

(3) To understand the advantages and disadvantages of solvent-free synthesis of metformin hydrochloride.

2   Introduction

The prevalence and incidences rate of diabetes are increasing worldwide. In addition, patients with diabetes may suffer from cardiovascular disease. Cardiovascular disease is the most important complication and major cause of death in diabetes patients worldwide. Nearly 60% of diabetes patients die from cardiovascular disease.

Metformin is a kind of oral hypoglycemic drug of biguanide. It is currently the first-line drug for treating diabetes mellitus type 2 worldwide. Metformin was launched in Europe in the 1950s, but it was not approved by the US FDA until December 30, 1994. Unlike sulfonylureas, metformin exhibits no effect on insulin secretion and does not stimulate islet β cells. No effect on blood glucose is observed in people without diabetes. The mechanism of antihyperglycemic includes reducing the absorption of glucose by the intestine, increasing the uptake of glucose from blood to tissue, reducing the production of glucose in the liver, and reducing the demand for insulin for glucose utilization. In addition, studies in recent years have also found that metformin shows a variety of pharmacological effects, such as improving blood lipids, regulating intestinal flora and human immunity, preventing and treating a variety of tumors, and even preventing aging and prolonging life at the animal level. New pharmacological effects of metformin are still being discovered and explored.

The method of synthesizing metformin hydrochloride mainly involves the nucleophilic addition reaction of dimethylamine hydrochloride to dicyandiamide. The reaction include solvent method and solvent-free method according to the reaction conditions. The solvent method is the main method of industrial synthesis. Due to the weak positive electricity of cyanide carbon in dicyandiamide, high boiling point solvents are often used as the medium, such as xylene and diphenyl ether, and water is also used as the solvent, and the reaction system is sealed under high pressure.

3   Experimental Principle

The solvent-free method is used in this experiment, and the reaction formula is shown in

Figure 4 – 1.

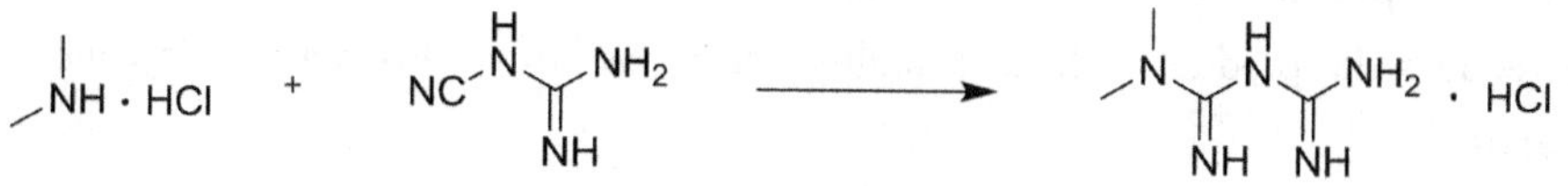

Figure 4 – 1   Synthesis of metformin hydrochloride

4   Experimental Procedure

4.1   Experimental Reagents

The experimental reagents are shown in Table 4 – 1.

Table 4 – 1   Dosage and specifications of experimental reagents

Reagents	Grade	Intended Amount	Amount of Substance/mmol	Molar Ratio	Safety Data
Dimethylamine hydrochloride	Analytical pure	2.45 g			
Dicyandiamide	Analytical pure	2.49 g			
95% Ethanol	Analytical pure	Approximately 20 mL/g crude product			

4.2   Method

2.45 g of dimethylamine hydrochloride and 2.49 g of dicyandiamide were added to the three-neck flask with a thermometer and a drying tube. The mixture was stirred and heated to 140 ℃ to melt the material. After the reactant solidified, the mixture continued to react for 1 h under the same conditions. After the reaction was stopped, approximately 20 mL of 95% ethanol was used to recrystallize each gram of crude product, and a large amount of white needle-like crystals was precipitated after standing. The crystals were filtered by suction and washed with 95% ethanol. The washed products were dried in an infrared rapid drying oven and weighed. The yield was calculated, and the melting point, infrared spectrum (IR) and ^{1}H-NMR were measured. (The reference yield is 40% – 60%, and the melting point of the purified product is 220 – 225 ℃.)

5   Notes

(1) When metformin hydrochloride is synthesized by the solvent-free method, with increasing reaction temperature, the time from melting state to reconversion to solid gradually shortens. For example, it takes approximately 100 min at 100 ℃, approximately 45 min at 120 ℃, and approximately 35 min at 140 ℃. However, it should be noted that when the temperature increases to more than 180 ℃, the compound may no longer be converted into a

solid. Through the reaction between products themselves and between products and raw materials, it is possible to generate a series of melamine derivatives (Figure 4 – 2), which greatly reduces the product yield and quality. Thus, the key to this reaction is controlling the temperature.

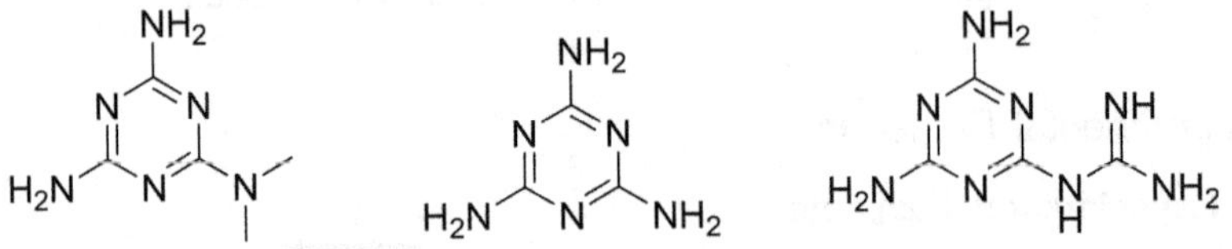

Figure 4 –2   Melamine derivatives

(2) In the recrystallization stage, the water content of ethanol shows a great influence on the solubility of metformin. For example, if 80% ethanol is used for recrystallization, only approximately 5 – 6 mL of solvent is needed for each gram of crude product, while approximately 40 mL solvent is needed for absolute ethanol.

6   Questions

(1) Review the literature and compare the advantages and disadvantages of solvent methods and solvent-free methods for the synthesis of metformin hydrochloride.

(2) Please discuss the mechanism of melamine impurities forming in the reaction of metformin synthesizing.

(3) If the solvent method is used for the reaction, which solvent (benzene, toluene or xylene) is more suitable for this reaction? What is the reason?

(4) Why does the reactant melt first and then solidify after the reaction continues?

(5) By comparing the IR and ^{1}H-NMR spectra of the product, which spectrum is easier to identify whether there is residual dicyandiamide?

实验五　苯妥英的合成

一、实验目的

（1）了解安息香缩合反应的原理和应用维生素 B_1 作为催化剂进行反应需要注意的操作。

（2）了解二苯羟乙酸重排反应机理。

（3）利用 $FeCl_3$ 作为氧化剂自行设计实验步骤制备二苯乙二酮。

（4）了解制备二苯乙二酮所采用的各种氧化方法的优缺点。

（5）巩固通过多步化学反应合成药物的思路与策略。

二、实验原理

苯妥英为经典抗癫痫药物，是药物化学课程重点介绍的药物之一。临床常用的是苯妥英的钠盐，即苯妥英钠。

苯妥英的合成（图 5-1）包含以下 3 个步骤：安息香缩合反应（安息香的制备），氧化反应（二苯乙二酮的制备），二苯羟乙酸重排及缩合反应（苯妥英的制备）。

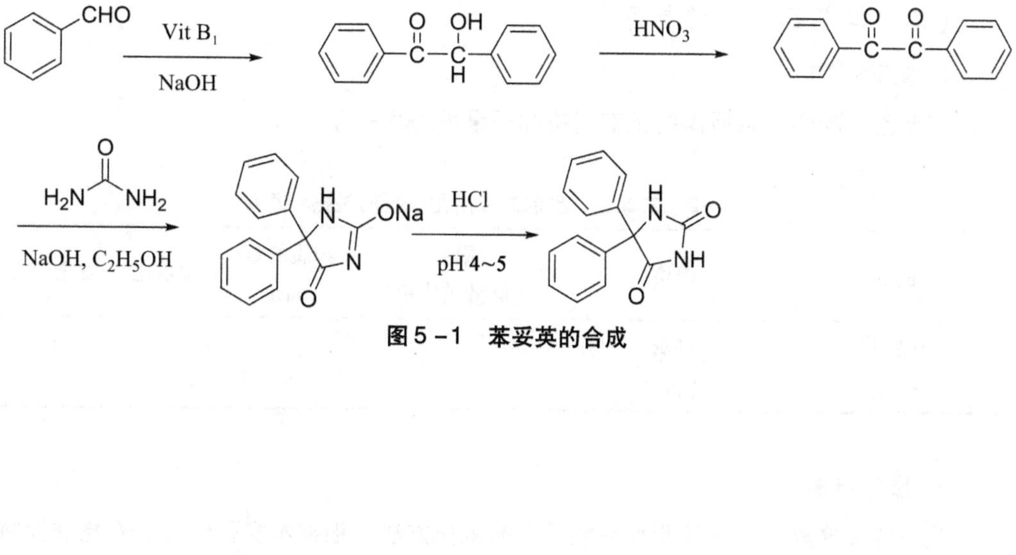

图 5-1　苯妥英的合成

三、实验方法

（一）安息香的制备

1. 实验试剂

安息香的制备所需试剂的规格和用量见表 5 – 1。

表 5 – 1　安息香制备所需实验试剂的规格和用量

试剂	规格	用量（重量或体积）	物质的量/mmol	摩尔比	安全信息
苯甲醛	分析纯	10 mL			
维生素 B_1	药用	1.7 g			
2 mol/L NaOH 溶液	—	5 mL			
95% 乙醇	分析纯	15 mL			

2. 操作步骤

在 100 mL 三口瓶中加入 1.7 g 维生素 B_1（硫胺素）和 4 mL 水，搅拌溶解后加入 95% 乙醇 15 mL。冰浴中冷却 10 min 后，搅拌下滴加 2 mol/L NaOH 溶液 5 mL。加完后，立即加入新蒸苯甲醛 10 mL，测 pH（pH > 8，没达到应补足）。水浴加热，65 ℃ 左右反应 1 h，再回流反应 30 min。冷却反应物至室温，析出大量晶体，冷水洗涤，抽干得到的粗品无须纯化，供下一步反应使用。测定产品熔点（参考熔点为 136 ～ 137 ℃）和 ^{1}H-NMR，TLC 检测纯度，计算产率。

（二）二苯乙二酮的制备

1. 实验试剂

二苯乙二酮的制备所需的试剂规格和用量见表 5 – 2。

表 5 – 2　二苯乙二酮的制备所需试剂的规格和用量

试剂	规格	用量（重量或体积）	物质的量/mmol	摩尔比	安全信息
安息香	自制	2.54 g			
$FeCl_3$	分析纯				

2. 操作步骤

通过查阅文献，了解该步反应能采用的氧化方法。根据本实验给出的安息香投料量，利用 FeCl$_3$ 作为氧化剂设计相应的实验步骤，合成二苯乙二酮。对比并讨论不同实验组采用不同实验操作和投料量对产物性状和产率的影响。测定产品熔点（参考熔点为 95～96 ℃）和 ^{1}H-NMR，TLC 检测纯度，计算产率。

（三）苯妥英的制备

1. 实验试剂

苯妥英的制备所需试剂的规格和用量见表 5－3。

表 5－3　苯妥英制备所需试剂的用量和规格

试剂	规格	用量（重量或体积）	物质的量/mmol	摩尔比	安全信息
二苯乙二酮	自制	2 g			
尿素	分析纯	0.75 g			
15% NaOH 溶液	—	6.3 mL			
95%乙醇	分析纯	10 mL			
15% HCl 溶液	—	适量			

2. 操作步骤

在装有搅拌及球形冷凝器的 100 mL 圆底瓶中，投入二苯乙二酮 2 g、尿素 0.75 g、15% NaOH 溶液 6.3 mL、95% 乙醇 10 mL，搅拌回流反应 60 min。反应完毕，将反应液倾入 65 mL 水中，搅拌后放置 15 min，抽滤以滤除黄色二苯乙炔二脲（图 5－2）沉淀。滤液用 15% HCl 溶液调至 pH＝6，放置，析出固体，抽滤，产物用少量水洗，得白色苯妥英粗品。如果产品颜色较深，应重新溶于碱液后，加活性炭煮沸 10 min 左右，冷却后，再酸化得白色针状结晶。测定产品熔点（参考熔点为 295～299 ℃）和 ^{1}H-NMR，TLC 检测纯度。

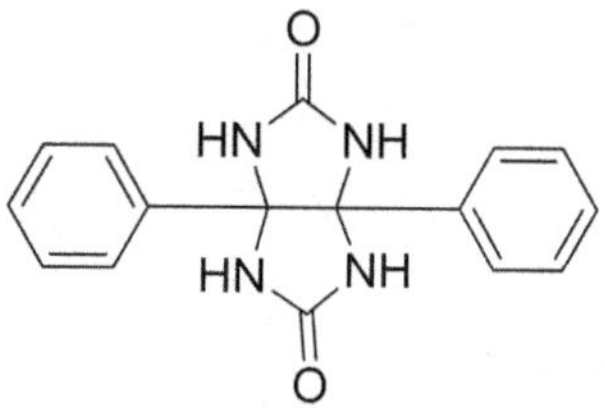

图 5－2　二苯乙炔二脲的结构式

四、附注

苯甲醛极易氧化，长期放置会有苯甲酸析出，本实验苯甲醛中不能含苯甲酸，因此用前须蒸馏。

五、思考题

（1）试述维生素 B_1 在安息香缩合反应中的作用（催化机理）。另外，还有什么催化剂常用于该类反应？为什么在本次安息香合成实验中不使用氰化钾作为催化剂？

（2）向维生素 B_1 中加入 NaOH 溶液前，为什么反应液需要预先冷却？

（3）在制备二苯乙二酮时，除使用 $FeCl_3$ 外，还有什么氧化方法可以选择？

（4）为什么制备苯妥英要在碱性条件下进行？

（5）对比并讨论不同实验组在用 $FeCl_3$ 制备二苯乙二酮过程中，不同实验操作和投料量对产物性状和产率的影响。

Experiment 5   Synthesis of Phenytoin

1   Learning Objectives

(1) To understand the principal of the benzoin condensation reaction and the operations that need to be observed when applying vitamin B_1 as a catalyst.

(2) To understand the principal of benzilic acid rearrangement reaction.

(3) Self-designed experimental steps for the preparation of benzil by ferric chloride as an oxidizing agent.

(4) To compare the advantages and disadvantages of various oxidation methods in the preparation of benzil.

(5) To learn the ideas and strategies for drug synthesis through multistep chemical reactions.

2   Experimental Principle

Phenytoin is a classic antiepileptic drug that was introduced in the course of medicinal chemistry. The sodium salt of phenytoin is commonly used in the clinic, namely, phenytoin sodium.

The synthesis of phenytoin (Figure 5 – 1) includes the following steps: a benzoin condensation reaction (preparation of benzoin); oxidation reaction (preparation of benzil); rearrangement of benzilic acid and condensation reaction (preparation of phenytoin).

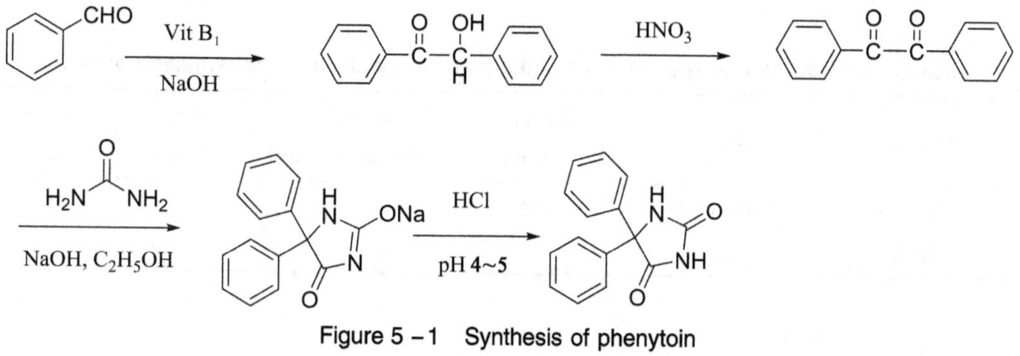

Figure 5 – 1   Synthesis of phenytoin

3   Experimental Procedure

3. 1   Synthesis of Benzoin

3. 1. 1   Experimental Reagents

The reagents required for the synthesis of benzoin are shown in Table 5 – 1.

Table 5 – 1　Dosage and specifications of the reagents required for the synthesis of benzoin

Reagents	Grade	Intended Amount	Amount of Substance/mmol	Molar Ratio	Safety Data
Benzaldehyde	Analytical pure	10 mL			
Vitamin B₁	Medical grade	1. 7 g			
2 mol/L NaOH solution	—	5 mL			
95% ethanol	Analytical pure	15 mL			

3. 1. 2　Method

1. 7 g of vitamin B_1 (thiamine hydrochloride) and 4 mL of water were added into a 100 mL three-neck flask and stirred to dissolve, and then 15 mL of 95% ethanol was added. After cooling in an ice bath for 10 min, 5 mL of 2 mol/L NaOH solution was added under stirring. After that, 10 mL of freshly evaporated benzaldehyde was added immediately, and the pH was measured (pH > 8, not achieved should be made up). The reaction was performed at 65 ℃ for 1 h and refluxed for 30 min. After cooling the reactants to room temperature, a large number of crystals were precipitated and then washed with cold water, and the crude product was dried without purification for the next reaction. The melting point (reference m. p. : 136 – 137 ℃) and ^{1}H-NMR of the product were determined. The purity was detected by TLC, and the yield of the product was calculated.

3. 2　Synthesis of Benzil

3. 2. 1　Experimental Reagents

The reagents required for the synthesis of benzil are shown in Table 5 – 2.

Table 5 – 2　Dosage and specifications of the reagents required for the synthesis of benzil

Reagents	Grade	Intended Amount	Amount of Substance/mmol	Molar Ratio	Safety Data
Benzoin	Home-made	2. 54 g			
FeCl₃	Analytical pure				

3. 2. 2　Method

Please investigate the oxidation methods that can be used for this step by consulting the literature. According to the amount of benzoin utilized in this experiment, design the corresponding experimental steps for the synthesis of benzil, using $FeCl_3$ chloride as the oxidizing agent. Compare and discuss the effects of different experimental operations and amounts on the product properties and yield. The product melting point (reference m. p. :

95 – 96 ℃) and ^{1}H-NMR were determined. The purity was detected by TLC, and the yield of the product was calculated.

3.3 Synthesis of Phenytoin

3.3.1 Experimental Reagents

The reagents required for the synthesis of phenytoin are shown in Table 5 – 3.

Table 5 –3   Dosage and specifications of the reagents required for the synthesis of phenytoin

Reagents	Grade	Intended Amount	Amount of Substance/mmol	Molar Ratio	Safety Data
Benzil	Home-made	2 g			
Urea	Analytical pure	0.75 g			
15% NaOH solution	—	6.3 mL			
95% Ethanol	95%	10 mL			
15% HCl solution	—	Appropriate amount			

3.3.2 Method

In a 100 mL round-bottom bottle with stirring, 2 g of benzil, 0.75 g of urea, 6.3 mL of 15% NaOH solution, and 10 mL of 95% ethanol were added. The reaction was refluxed for 60 min. Then, the reactant was poured into 65 mL of water and stirred. After standing for 15 min, the mixture was filtered to remove the yellow impurities diphenylacetylene diurea (Figure 5 –2). The yellow impurities were filtered out. The filtrate was adjusted to pH = 6 with 15% HCl, and the precipitated solids were placed and filtered. The product was washed with a small amount of water to obtain white crude phenytoin. If the product color is darker, the product should be redissolved in alkali and boiled with activated carbon for approximately 10 min. After cooling, the product should be acidified to obtain white needle crystals. The melting point (reference m.p.: 295 – 299 ℃) and ^{1}H-NMR of the product were determined, and the purity was detected by TLC.

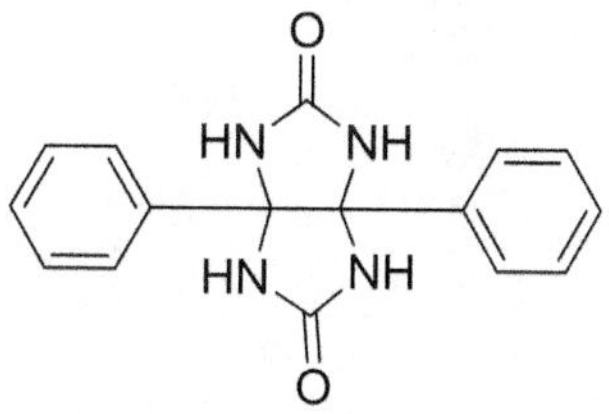

Figure 5 –2   The structural formula of diphenylacetylene diurea

4   Notes

Benzaldehyde is easily oxidized, and benzoic acid is precipitated when placed for a long time. In this experiment, benzaldehyde could not contain benzoic acid, so it must be distilled before use.

5 Questions

(1) Describe the role of vitamin B_1 in the condensation reaction of benzoin (catalytic mechanism). In addition, what other catalysts are commonly used for this kind of reaction? Why is potassium cyanide not used as a catalyst in this experiment?

(2) Before NaOH solution is added to vitamin B_1, why does the reaction solution need to be precooled?

(3) In addition to using $FeCl_3$, what other oxidation methods are available when preparing benzil?

(4) Why is the preparation of phenytoin carried out under alkaline conditions?

(5) Compare and discuss the effects of different experimental operations and amounts on the product properties and yield in the process of preparing benzil with $FeCl_3$.

实验六　双氢青蒿素的合成

一、实验目的

（1）了解各种还原试剂的性质和适用范围。

（2）掌握 KBH_4 还原反应的注意事项。

（3）了解青蒿素作为抗疟疾药物的发现过程及发展。

二、背景知识

据世界卫生组织统计，全球每年因疟疾感染而导致死亡的人数为 100 万至 200 万，其中一半以上为 5 岁以下的儿童。近一个世纪以来，里程碑式的抗疟药共有 3 个，即 1945 年的氯喹、1985 年的甲氟喹、1987 年的青蒿素类衍生物，前两个因为耐药性的产生在临床上已经较少使用，而青蒿素（artemisinin）（图 6 - 1 和图 6 - 2）及其衍生物是目前最有效的抗疟药。青蒿素（CAS 63968-64-9），化学名称为（3R，5aS，6R，8aS，9R，12S，12aR）- 八氢 - 3，6，9 - 三甲基 - 3，12 - 氧桥 - 12H - 吡喃并［4，3-j］- 1，2 - 苯并二塞平 - 10（3H）- 酮，分子式为 $C_{15}H_{22}O_5$，熔点为 151～153 ℃，属倍半萜内酯类化合物，具有过氧键和内酯环结构，这一结构在天然产物中十分罕见。1971 年，中国药学家屠呦呦在植物黄花蒿茎叶的乙醚提取液中分离纯化得到青蒿素，并证实其为新型高效抗疟疾药物，尤其是对于脑型疟疾和抗氯喹疟疾，具有速效和低毒的特点，在临床中拯救了数百万人的生命。屠呦呦因此获得 2011 年的拉斯克临床医学研究奖和 2015 年诺贝尔生理学或医学奖。

临床使用中发现青蒿素具有口服活性低、溶解度小、生物利用度低、半衰期短、复发率高等不足。因此，需要对青蒿素进行化学修饰以开发更适用于临床使用的药物，过氧桥结构是青蒿素发挥抗疟活性的关键结构单元，对青蒿素结构进行修饰和改造时应保留该结构。目前临床广泛应用的双氢青蒿素（图 6 - 3）、蒿甲醚（图 6 - 4）和青蒿琥酯（图 6 - 5）都保留了三氧杂环己烷骨架。

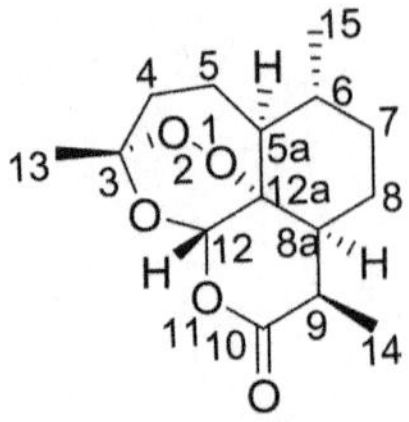

图 6-1 青蒿素

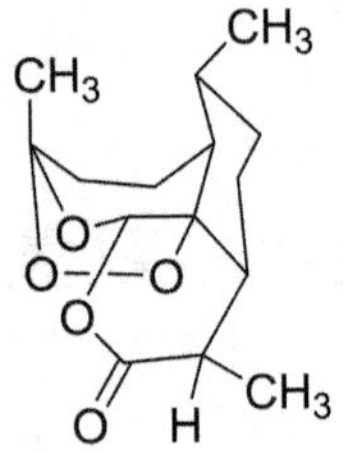

图 6-2 青蒿素的立体构型

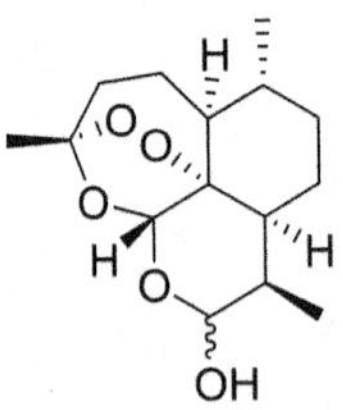

图 6-3 双氢青蒿素

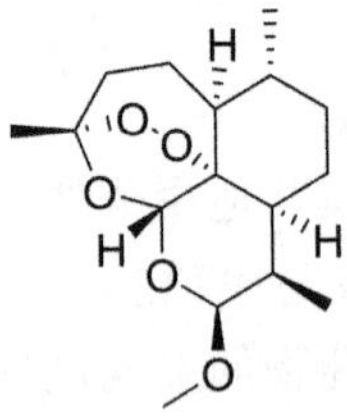

图 6-4 蒿甲醚

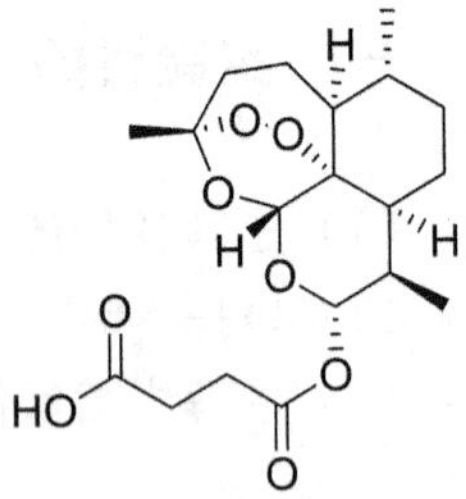

图 6-5 青蒿琥酯

双氢青蒿素（dihydroartemisinin），分子式为 $C_{15}H_{24}O_5$，根据 10 - 位构型不同，有 α（10 R，CAS 81496-81-3）和 β（10 S，CAS 71939-50-9）两种差向异构体，其化学名为（3R，5aS，6R，8aS，9R，10S，12R，12aR）- 八氢 -3，6，9 - 三甲基 -3，12 - 桥氧 -12 H - 吡喃并［4，3-j］-1，2 - 苯并二噻平 -10（3H）- 醇。双氢青蒿素是青蒿素类药物在体内的主要活性代谢产物，活性约为青蒿素的 2 倍，与青蒿素相比生物利用度略有提高且更易吸收，具有排泄和代谢迅速、高效、低毒等优点，但结构不太稳定，目前主要作为合成其他青蒿素衍生物的中间体。通常由 $NaBH_4$ 还原青蒿素得到，最初得到的产品以 β 构型（图 6-6）为主，在溶液中会缓慢转化为 α 构型（图 6-7），最终达到平衡，在室温甲醇溶液中平衡后 α : β ≈ 2 : 1，酸和加热会极大促进这种平衡的进行，转化速率常数和平衡常数与溶剂的质子传递能力成正相关。α 构型异构体的极性比 β 构型异构体的大，因为它的—OH 与过氧桥在同一侧。β 构型异构体在甲醇中的溶解度要小于 α 构型异构体，可用甲醇为重结晶溶剂纯化 β 构型异构体。

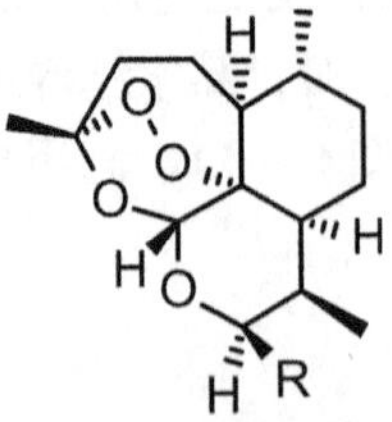

图 6-6 β 构型双氢青蒿素

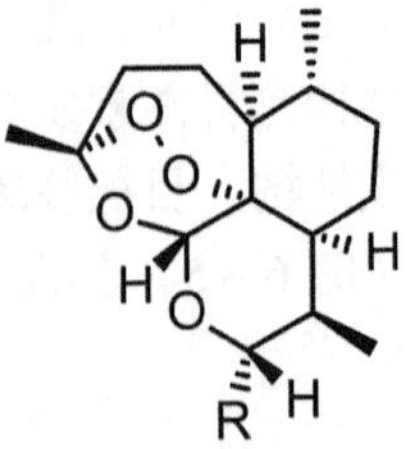

图 6-7 α 构型双氢青蒿素

三、实验原理

双氢青蒿素合成的实验原理如图 6 – 8 所示。

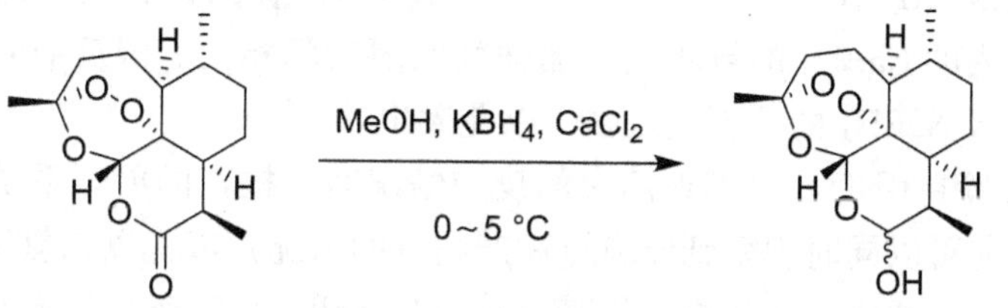

MeOH, KBH$_4$, CaCl$_2$

0~5 ℃

图 6 – 8　双氢青蒿素的合成

四、实验方法

（一）实验试剂

实验用试剂规格和用量见表 6 – 1。

表 6 – 1　双氢青蒿素合成所需试剂的规格和用量

试剂	规格	用量 （重量或体积）	物质的量/ mmol	摩尔比	安全信息
青蒿素	药用	0.50 g			
无水甲醇	分析纯	5 mL			
KBH$_4$	分析纯	0.38 g			
无水 CaCl$_2$	分析纯	0.10 g			
乙醇	分析纯	适量			

（二）操作步骤

在 50 mL 干燥的圆底烧瓶中加入 0.50 g 青蒿素，再加入 5 mL 无水甲醇和 0.10 g 粉状无水 CaCl$_2$，5 ℃ 冰水浴下搅拌，分 2 次加入 0.38 g KBH$_4$，每次 0.19 g，间隔 5 min，在 5 ℃ 冰水浴下继续搅拌 1 h，通过 TLC 监测反应进程，至原料青蒿素消失（一般需 45 ~ 60 min）。反应结束后，在冰浴下用乙酸中和反应液至 pH = 6，加入冷水（5 倍体积，25 mL），冰浴搅拌 10 min，抽滤，冰水洗涤，滤饼经红外干燥得白色固体。参考收率为 70% ~ 80%，粗品熔点为 142 ~ 148 ℃。不纯的产品可用 10 ~ 20 倍量无水乙醇重结晶，干燥，得白色固体，重结晶回收率约为 90%，精品熔点为 145 ~ 150 ℃。

五、附注

（1）与 $NaBH_4$ 相比，KBH_4 还原活性低一些，但是 KBH_4 不易吸潮，更容易操作。如果采用 $NaBH_4$ 作还原剂的话，要注意防止称量过程吸潮，最好分多次称量，尽量使每批加入的 $NaBH_4$ 的量相同、加样的间隔时间相同。因反应时会放出大量气泡，固每次加入 $NaBH_4$ 的量不宜过多，以免溢出。

（2）本实验在用 TLC 检测青蒿素的反应情况时，推荐的展开系统为石油醚：乙酸乙酯 = 4∶1（可以同时观察到原料点和产物点的情况）或先以二氯甲烷展开，观察原料是否有剩余，再以二氯甲烷：甲醇 = 30∶1 展开，观察产品。不同的硅胶板薄层情况可能有所不同，应根据初始的薄层结果对展开剂极性进行适当的调整。

六、思考题

（1）请查阅文献，试述当采用其他类型的还原剂还原青蒿素的时候，所得到的产物有何不同？

（2）$CaCl_2$ 在该反应中的作用是什么？

（3）反应结束后加酸调 pH 的目的是什么？

（4）反应结束后加水处理样品的目的是什么？

（5）如何通过 ^1H-NMR 来判断青蒿素和双氢青蒿素？

Experiment 6　Synthesis of Dihydroartemisinin

1　Learning Objectives

(1) To understand the properties and applications of reductants.

(2) To master reduction reactions with potassium borohydride.

(3) To understand the discovery and development of artemisinin as an antimalarial drug.

2　Introduction

According to the statistics provided by the WHO, 1 million to 2 million global deaths are attributed to malaria infection each year, and more than half of the deaths occur in children under 5 years of age. In nearly a century, 3 milestone antimalarial drugs were discovered, namely, chloroquine in 1945, mefloquine in 1985, and artemisinin derivatives in 1987. The first two, however, were less applied to the clinic due to drug tolerance. Artemisinin (Figure 6 – 1 and Figure 6 – 2) and its derivatives remain the most effective antimalarial drugs. Artemisinin (CAS 63968-64-9), which is chemically named (3R, 5aS, 6R, 8aS, 9R, 12S, 12aR) -octahydro-3, 6, 9-trimethyl-3, 12-epoxy-12 H-pyrano[4, 3-j] -1, 2-benzodioxepin-10 (3 H) -one, molecular formula $C_{15}H_{22}O_5$, m. p. 151 – 153 ℃, is a sesquiterpene lactone compound consisting of peroxy bonds and lactonic ring structures, which are rather rare among natural products. In 1971, artemisinin was first separated from the diethyl ether extract of plant *Artemisia annua* stems and leaves by the Chinese pharmaceutical chemist Tu Youyou. Subsequently, artemisinin was proved as a novel effective antimalarial drug, especially for cerebral malaria and chloroquine-resistant malaria, with high efficiency and low toxicity. Tu Youyou was therefore honored with the Lasker-DeBakey Clinical Medical Research Award in 2011 and the Nobel Prize in Physiology or Medicine 2015 for saving millions of lives in clinical practice.

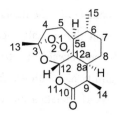

Figure 6 – 1　Artemisinin

Figure 6 – 2　Three-dimensional structure of artemisinin

At clinical application, it was found that artemisinin involves drawbacks, such as low activity with oral administration, low solubility, low bioavailability, short half-life and high relapse rate. Therefore, Chemical modification was applied to artemisinin for the development of novel drugs that are more suitable for clinical applications. The peroxo bridge is the key moiety for the antimalarial activity of artemisinin. Therefore, the modification of the artemisinin structure have resulted in dihydroartemisinin (Figure 6 – 3), artemether (Figure 6 – 4), and artesunate (Figure 6 – 5), which are widely used in clinical practice. The compounds all retain the trioxane skeleton.

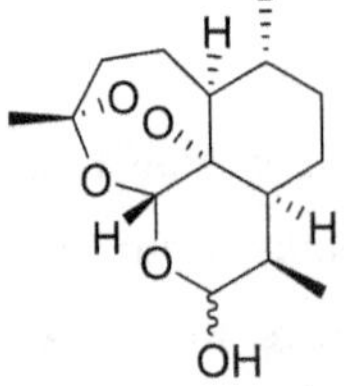

Figure 6 – 3   Dihydroar-
temisinin

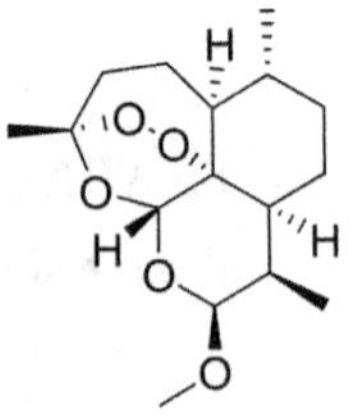

Figure 6 – 4   Artemether

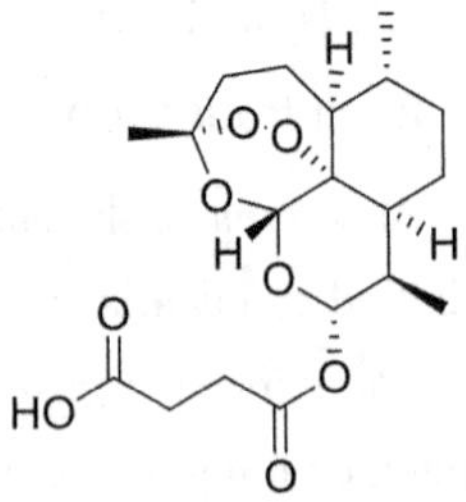

Figure 6 – 5   Artesunate

Dihydroartemisinin (molecular formula: $C_{15}H_{24}O_5$) has two isomers of α (10R, CAS 81 496-81-3) and β (10S, CAS 71939-50-9) according to the C-10 configuration, which is chemically named (3R, 5aS, 6R, 8aS, 9R, 10S, 12R, 12aR) -decahydro-3, 6, 9-trimethyl-3, 12-epoxy-12H-pyrano [4, 3-j] -1, 2-benzodioxepin-10 (3H) -ol. Dihydroartemisinin is the main active metabolite of artemisinins, with an activity approximately twice as good as that of artemisinin. Compared to artemisinin, dihydroartemisinin exhibits several advantages, including slightly higher bioavailability, easier absorption, faster excretion and metabolism, higher efficiency and lower toxicity. However, the structure of dihydroartemisinin is rather unstable. Currently, the compound mainly serves as an intermediate for the synthesis of other artemisinin derivatives. Dihydroartemisinin is usually obtained by the reduction of artemisinin by $NaBH_4$. The initial products are mainly β-isomers (Figure 6 – 6), which gradually transform into α-isomers(Figure 6 – 7) and finally reach a balance. In methanol solution at room temperature, the balance is $\alpha : \beta \approx 2 : 1$. Acidity and heat dramatically accelerate the process of reaching a balance, and there is a positive correlation between the transition rate constants and equilibrium constants with the proton transfer ability of solutions. The α-isomer exhibits higher polarity than that of the β-isomer since its – OH moieties are on the same side as the peroxo bridge. Compared to the α-isomer, the β-isomer shows lower solubility in methanol, and therefore, methanol can be used as the recrystallization solution for β-isomer purification.

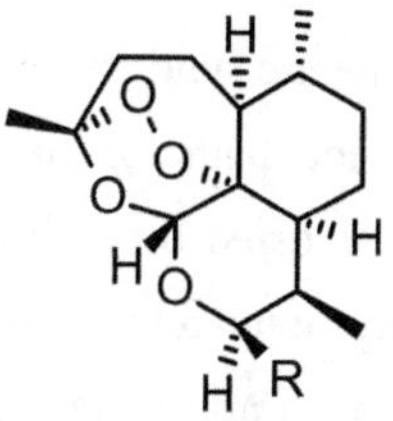

Figure 6 – 6　α-Isomer

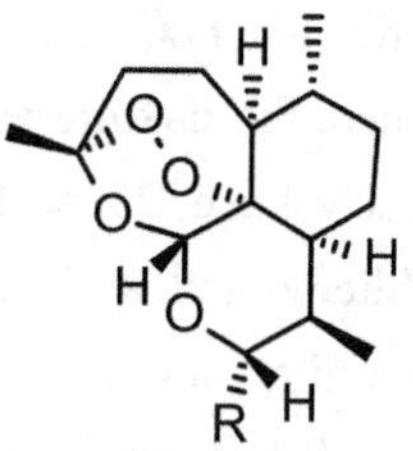

Figure 6 – 7　β-Isomer

3　Experimental Principle

The synthesis of dihydroartemisinin is shown in Figure 6 – 8.

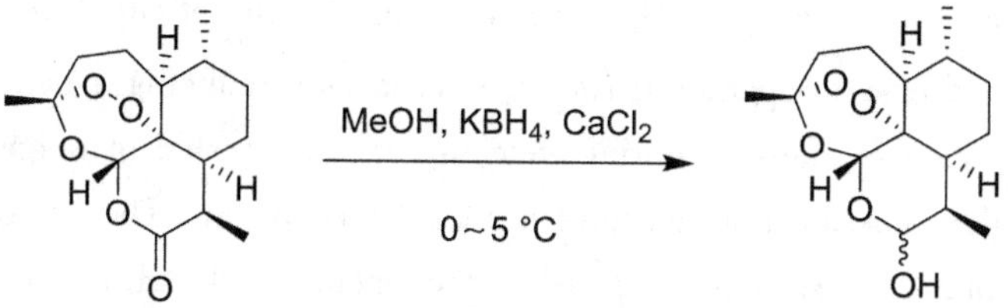

Figure 6 – 8　Synthesis of dihydroartemisinin

4　Experimental Procedure

4.1　Experimental Reagents

The experimental reagents are shown in Table 6 – 1.

Table 6 – 1　Dosage and specifications of experimental reagents

Reagents	Grade	Intended Amount	Amount of Substance/mmol	Molar Ratio	Safety Data
Artemisinin	Medical grade	0.50 g			
Methanol	Analytical pure	5 mL			
KBH_4	Analytical pure	0.38 g			
$CaCl_2$	Analytical pure	0.10 g			
Acetic acid	Analytical pure	appropriate amount			

4.2　Method

0.50 g of artemisinin was added to a dry 50 mL round-bottom flask, and then 5 mL of anhydrous methanol and 0.10 g of powdered anhydrous $CaCl_2$ were added. The mixture was stirred in an ice water bath at 5 ℃. 0.38 g of KBH_4 was added twice, 0.19 g each time, with an interval of 5 min. The mixture was stirred in an ice water bath at 5 ℃, and the progress was monitored with TLC until artemisinin disappeared (usually 45 – 60 min). After the reaction finished, the mixture was neutralized to pH = 6 with acetic acid in an ice bath. Cold water (5 times volume, 25 mL) was added and stirred in an ice bath for 10 min. The solid residue was filtered and washed with ice water. The residue was dried through infrared drying and afforded white solid products. The reference yield is approximately 70% – 80%. The melting point of the crude product is 142 – 148 ℃. The impure products could be recrystallized with 10 – 20 times the volume of ethanol(v/w). The mixture was dried to obtain white solid product. The yield of recrystallization is approximately 90%. The melting point of the purified product is 145 – 150 ℃.

5 Notes

(1) Compared with $NaBH_4$, KBH_4 has lower reducing in activity. However, KBH_4 is not easy to moisten and easy to operate. If $NaBH_4$ is used as a reducing agent, it is necessary to prevent the absorption of moisture during weighing. It is suggested to weigh $NaBH_4$ multiple times and keep the same amount and interval time for each time. The reaction will release a large number of bubbles, and to avoid overflow, the amount of $NaBH_4$ should not be added too much at a time.

(2) When using TLC to monitor the reaction of artemisinin in this experiment, the suggested eluent is petroleum ether : ethyl acetate = 4 : 1 (spots of the raw material and product can be observed at the same time) or dichloromethane for the first time to observe any raw material that remain, then separate should be performed with dichloromethane : methanol = 30: 1 to observe the products. Notice that the cases might be different depending on the silica gel plates, so the polarity of the developing solvent should be appropriately adjusted according to the initial TLC results.

6 Questions

(1) Please consult the literature. What are the differences of products when other types of reducing agents are used to reduce artemisinin?

(2) What is the role of $CaCl_2$ in this reaction?

(3) What is the purpose of adjusting the pH with acid after the reaction is finished?

(4) What is the purpose of treating the samples by adding water?

(5) How to distinguish artemisinin or dihydroartemisinin by ^{1}H-NMR?

实验七 蒿甲醚的合成

一、实验目的

（1）了解蒿甲醚的发现过程及其在抗疟治疗中的应用。
（2）掌握蒿甲醚合成的常用方法、原理及优缺点。

二、背景知识

蒿甲醚（artemether，CAS 71963-77-4），分子式为 $C_{16}H_{26}O_5$，化学名为（3R，5aS，6R，8aS，9R，10S，12R，12aR）－十氢－10－甲氧基－3，6，9－三甲基－3，12－桥氧－12H－吡喃并［4，3-j］－1，2－苯并二噻平，是由青蒿素经甲醚化而成。蒿甲醚在体外的稳定性及抗疟活性较双氢青蒿素都有显著提高，其具有水溶性差、脂溶性好的特点，便于制成油剂给药，其在体内快速代谢为双氢青蒿素起作用。蒿甲醚的抗疟活性是青蒿素的 3～7 倍，产物一般以 β 构型为主，但 α 和 β 差向异构体的活性没有太大差别，现广泛用于临床治疗疟疾。

三、实验原理

蒿甲醚的合成如图 7－1 所示。

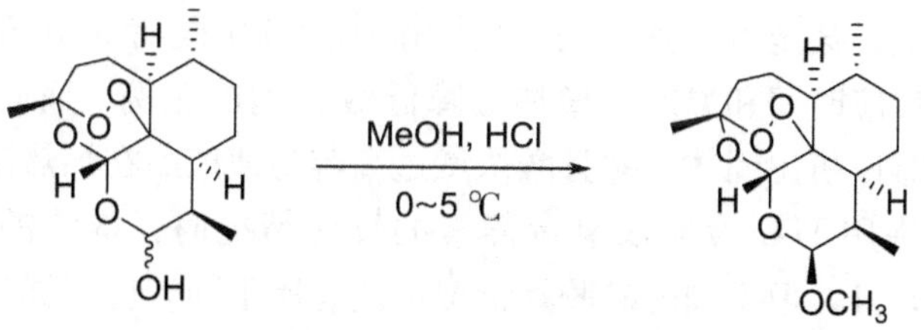

图 7－1　蒿甲醚的合成

四、实验方法

（一）原料规格及配比

1. 实验试剂

实验用试剂的规格和用量见表 7 - 1。

表 7 - 1　蒿甲醚合成所需试剂的规格和用量

试剂	规格	用量（重量或体积）	物质的量/mmol	摩尔比	安全信息
双氢青蒿素	药用	0.50 g			
甲醇	分析纯	20 mL			
浓 HCl	分析纯	1～2 滴			

（二）操作步骤

在干燥的 50 mL 圆底烧瓶中加入双氢青蒿素 0.50 g 和甲醇 20 mL，室温搅拌溶解后加入浓 HCl 1～2 滴。继续在室温下搅拌反应，通过 TLC 监测反应进程至原料双氢青蒿素消失（2～3 h）。反应结束后，减压蒸除溶剂，加入冰冷的甲醇/水溶液 6 mL（甲醇：水 = 1：2，v/v），冰浴搅拌 10 min 以上。抽滤，用甲醇/水溶液（甲醇：水 = 1：2，u/v）洗涤，滤饼真空干燥，得到白色固体，参考收率为 40%～60%。用柱层析进行纯化得到白色固体，柱层析回收率为 40%～50%，熔点为 85～87 ℃。

五、附注

（1）在本实验中，加入酸的量是蒿甲醚合成反应的关键，加入过量的酸会使实验失败或收率降低，甚至得不到产物。反应生成的蒿甲醚有 α 和 β 两种构型。溶剂极性、酸浓度、反应时间和温度的增加会降低 β 构型的比例，而 α 构型的增加会导致后处理的时候难以析出固体，并且酸浓度过高容易使产品在加热浓缩时分解。

（2）本实验在用 TLC 检测双氢青蒿素的反应情况时，推荐的展开系统为石油醚：乙酸乙酯 = 4：1，但不同的硅胶板情况可能有所不同，应根据初始的薄层色谱结果对展开剂极性进行适当的调整。β 构型的极性略低于 α 构型。在本反应体系中以 β 构型为主，β：α = 4：1～3：2。

（3）在进行减压蒸馏时，温度设定不能超过 40 ℃，因为蒿甲醚熔点低，并且不宜蒸得过干。减压蒸除溶剂时，若温度过高，会使蒿甲醚熔化和分解变色（浅紫色至深褐色），对后处理造成困难。

（4）如果加入甲醇/水溶液后立即有大量白色固体析出，则冰浴中搅拌 10 min 后即可抽滤；如果得到的是油状黏性液体，可加入多一倍的甲醇/水溶液，并需要较长时间的搅拌处理。

（5）干燥时最好使用真空干燥或冷冻干燥，由于产品熔点低，使用红外干燥或烘箱干燥容易导致产品熔化。

（6）本实验在用柱层析对反应产物进行纯化时，推荐的洗脱系统为石油醚∶乙酸乙酯＝10∶1，但不同品牌和粒度的硅胶情况可能有所不同，应根据初始的薄层色谱结果对洗脱液极性进行适当的调整。

六、思考题

（1）查阅文献，分析本实验主要的副产物是什么，什么原因导致了该副产物的产生？

（2）查阅文献，试述合成蒿甲醚时，所采用的酸还有哪些？各有哪些优缺点？

（3）原料双氢青蒿素与产物蒿甲醚在 IR 和 ^{1}H-NMR 图谱中最大的差别表现在哪里？请讨论。

Experiment 7   Synthesis of Artemether

1   Learning Objectives

(1) To understand the discovery of artemether and its application in antimalarial treatments.

(2) To master the common methods, principles, advantages and disadvantages of artemether synthesis.

2   Introduction

Artemether (CAS 71963-77-4), molecular formula $C_{16}H_{26}O_5$, which is chemically named (3R, 5aS, 6R, 8aS, 9R, 10S, 12R, 12aR)-decahydro-10-methoxy-3, 6, 9-trimethyl-3, 12-epoxy-12H-pyrano (4, 3-j)-1, 2-benzodioxepin, is obtained from the methoxylation of artemisinin. The stability and antimalarial activity of artemether *in vitro* are remarkably improved compared with those of artemisinin. Artemether exhibits poor water solubility and good lipid solubility; thus, artemether can be converted into an oil agent, which is convenient to administer and provides rapid effects through metabolism into dihydroartemisinin *in vivo*. Artemether shows 3 – 7 times better antimalarial activity than that of artemisinin. The products are mainly β-isomers, although there is no significant difference between the α-isomers and β-isomers, and the products are widely used for clinical malaria therapies.

3   Experimental Principle

The synthesis of artemether is shown in Figure 7 – 1.

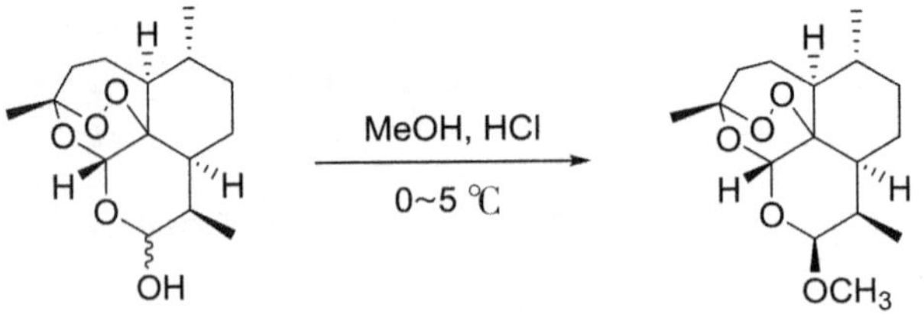

Figure 7 – 1   Synthesis of artemether

4 Experimental Procedure

4.1 Experimental Reagents

The experimental reagents are shown in Table 7 – 1.

Table 7 – 1 Dosage and specifications of experimental reagents

Reagents	Grade	Intended Amount	Amount of Substance/mmol	Molar Ratio	Safety Data
Dihydroartemisinin	Medical grade	0.50 g			
Methanol	Analytical pure	20 mL			
Concentrated HCl	Analytical pure	1 – 2 Drops			

4.2 Method

0.50 g of Dihydroartemisinin was added to a dry 50 mL round-bottom flask and dissolved in 20 mL of methanol by stirring at room temperature. Then, 1 – 2 drops of concentrated HCl solution were added. The mixture was stirred at room temperature, and the progress of the reaction was monitored with TLC until dihydroartemisinin disappeared (2 – 3 h). After the reaction was finished, the solvent was evaporated under reduced pressure, and then 6 mL of cold methanol/water solution (methanol: water = 1:2, v/v) was added and stirred in an ice bath for more than 10 min. The white solid was obtained by filtration and washing with methanol/water solution (methanol: water = 1:2, v/v), and the solid residue was dried under vacuum. The reference yield is 40% – 60%. The white solid was obtained by purification with column chromatography. The reference yield of column chromatography is 40% – 50%. The product m. p. is 85 – 87 ℃.

5 Notes

(1) In this experiment, the calculated amount is the key to the synthesis of artemether. Notably, adding excessive acid will lead to the failure of the experiment or the decrement of the yield, or even no products are obtained. The yielded artemether products contain two differential isomers, α-isomer and β-isomer. The increment of the solvent polarity, acid concentration, reaction time and temperature will lower the proportion of the β-isomer and the increase of α-isomer will make it difficult to precipitate solids during post-processing. Moreover, during the process of heating and concentrating, excessively high acidic concentration may lead to product decomposition.

(2) When monitoring the progress of the dihydroartemisinin reaction with TLC, the recommended eluent system is petroleum ether : ethyl acetate = 4 : 1. However, different thin layers of silica gel plate may produce different results. The polarity of the developing solvent should be adjusted according to the initial thin layer results. The β-isomer shows a slightly

lower polarity than that of the α-isomer, and the β-isomer is the main configuration in this reaction system (β : α = 4 : 1 - 3 : 2).

(3) During vacuum distillation, the temperature setting should not be over 40 ℃ because artemether has a low melting point, and it is not recommended to completely dry out the products. When evaporating the solvent, the products will be melted and decomposed with color changes (light purple to dark brown) if the temperature is too high, causing difficulties in the work up.

(4) Once the methanol/water solution is added, if a large amount of white solids participate, the mixture can be filtered after being stirred in ice bath for 10 min. However, if oily products are obtained, another volume of methanol/water solution can be added, and the mixture is stirred for a longer time.

(5) It is recommended to use vacuum drying or freeze drying when drying the products due to its low melting point. Infrared drying or oven drying will likely to cause the product melting.

(6) When purifying the products with column chromatography in this experiment, the recommended eluent is petroleum ether : ethyl acetate = 10 : 1. However, there might be differences in the brands and particle sizes of the silica gel, so the eluent polarity should be adjusted according to the initial TLC results.

6 Questions

(1) Referring to the literature, please analyze the main byproducts in this experiment and what causes the byproducts.

(2) Referring to the literature, please determine what other acids can be used in artemether synthesis and what the advantages and disadvantages of these acids are.

(3) Please discuss what is the most significant difference between the ingredient dihydroartemisinin and the product artemether in the IR and H-NMR spectra.

实验八　青蒿琥酯的合成

一、实验目的

（1）掌握青蒿琥酯的设计原理。
（2）了解青蒿琥酯在临床中的特殊应用。

二、背景知识

青蒿琥酯（artesunate，CAS 88495-63-0），分子式为 $C_{19}H_{28}O_8$，化学名为 1 - ［(3R，5aS，6R，8aS，9R，10S，12R，12aR) - 十氢 - 3，6，9 - 三甲基 - 3，12 - 桥氧 - 12H - 吡喃并［4，3-j］ - 1，2 - 苯并二塞平 - 10 醇］ - 丁二酸酯，是由双氢青蒿素酯化而成，是单一的 α 异构体，也是第一个水溶性青蒿素衍生物，其抗疟活性是青蒿素的 3～7 倍，适用于注射给药，急性和亚急性毒性低，常用于凶险型疟疾的急救。

三、实验原理

青蒿琥酯的合成如图 8 -1 所示。

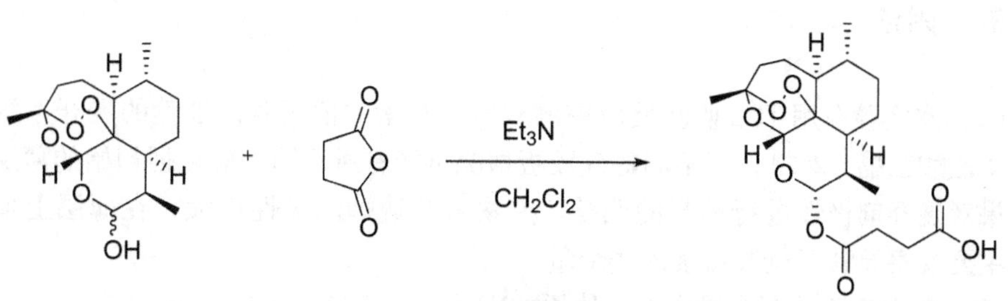

图 8 -1　青蒿琥酯的合成

四、实验方法

(一) 实验试剂

青蒿琥酯合成所需试剂的规格及用量见表 8 - 1。

表 8 - 1　青蒿琥酯合成所需试剂的规格及用量

试剂	规格	用量（重量或体积）	物质的量/mmol	摩尔比	安全信息
双氢青蒿素	药用	0.50 g			
二氯甲烷	分析纯	5 mL			
丁二酸酐	分析纯	0.35 g			
三乙胺	分析纯	0.25 mL			
0.2 mol/L H$_2$SO$_4$ 溶液	—	20 mL			
无水硫酸钠	分析纯	适量			

(二) 操作步骤

称取双氢青蒿素 0.50 g 于 50 mL 圆底烧瓶中，加入 5 mL 二氯甲烷、0.35 g 丁二酸酐和 0.25 mL 三乙胺，室温密闭搅拌反应，通过 TLC 监测反应进程，直至原料双氢青蒿素消失（通常需 2～2.5 h）。反应结束后，加入二氯甲烷 25 mL 和 0.2 mol/L H$_2$SO$_4$ 溶液 20 mL，置分液漏斗中萃取，使水层和有机层分离，用水洗涤有机层 2 次后将有机层收集起来。用无水 Na$_2$SO$_4$ 干燥收集有机层，过滤，减压浓缩得白色固体，参考收率为 80%～85%，熔点为 132～135 ℃。

五、附注

（1）本实验在用 TLC 监测反应中的双氢青蒿素的情况时，推荐的展开系统为石油醚：乙酸乙酯 = 2 : 1，但不同的硅胶板情况可能有所不同，应根据初始的薄层色谱法结果对展开剂极性进行适当的调整。产物青蒿琥酯的极性很大，在薄层上拖尾严重，主要观察原料双氢青蒿素的残余量。

（2）在本实验的萃取操作中，使用的 H$_2$SO$_4$ 溶液浓度不宜过高。

（3）如果得到黏性较大的固体，可适当放置一段时间，然后用玻棒摩擦搅拌，这有助于固体的转化。

六、思考题

（1）如何通过萃取的方法，在反应混合物的后处理中除去未反应的双氢青蒿素？

（2）该实验采用三乙胺作为碱，请问是否可以采用 NaOH 代替三乙胺？

（3）原料双氢青蒿素与产物青蒿琥酯在 IR 和[1]H-NMR 图谱中最大的差别表现在哪里？请讨论。

Experiment 8   Synthesis of Artesunate

1   Learning Objectives

(1) To master the design principle of artesunate.

(2) To understand the special clinical application of artesunate.

2   Introduction

Artesunate (CAS 88495-63-0) (molecular formula $C_{19} H_{28} O_8$), chemical named Butanedioic acid, 1-[($3R, 5aS, 6R, 8aS, 9R, 10S, 12R, 12aR$) -decahydro-3, 6, 9-trimethyl-3, 12-epoxy-12H-pyrano [4, 3-j] -1, 2-benzodioxepin-10-yl] ester, is obtained from the esterification of dihydroartemisinin. Artesunate only has single α-isomer, and it is the first water-soluble artemisinin analog. Artesunate exhibits antimalarial activity 3 − 7 times stronger than that of artemisinin, and it is suitable for injection administration. It also shows low acute and subacute toxicity and is often used in first aid for dangerous malaria.

3   Experimental Principle

The synthesis of artesunate is shown in Figure 8 − 1.

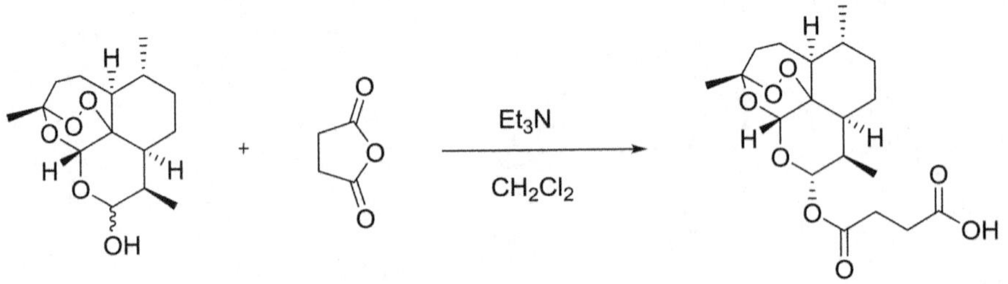

Figure 8 − 1   Synthesis of artesunate

4   Experimental Procedure

4. 1   Experimental Reagents

The experimental reagents are shown in Table 8 − 1.

Table 8 − 1   Dosage and specifications of experimental reagents

Reagents	Grade	Intended Amount	Amount of Substance/mmol	Molar Ratio	Safety Data
Dihydroartemisinin	Medical grade	0. 50 g			
Dichloromethane	Analytical pure	5 mL			

Table 8 – 1 （Continued）

Reagents	Grade	Intended Amount	Amount of Substance/mmol	Molar Ratio	Safety Data
Succinic anhydride	Analytical pure	0. 35 g			
Triethylamine	Analytical pure	0. 25 mL			
0. 2 mol/L H$_2$SO$_4$ solution	—	20 mL			
Anhydrous sodium sulfate	Analytical pure	Appropriate amount			

4. 2　Method

0. 50 g of dihydroartemisinin was added to a 50 mL round-bottom flask, and 5 mL of dichloromethane, 0. 35 g of succinic anhydride and 0. 25 mL of triethylamine were added, the flask was sealed and the reaction was stirred at room temperature. The reaction progress was monitored with TLC until the dihydroartemisinin disappeared (generally 2 – 2. 5 h). After the reaction, 25 mL of dichloromethane and 20 mL of 0. 2 mol/L H$_2$SO$_4$ solution were added and extracted in the separating funnel to separate the water layer and the organic layer. The organic layer was washed twice with water and then collected. The product was dried with anhydrous sodium sulfate, filtered, and concentrated under reduced pressure to obtain a white solid. The reference yield was 80% – 85%, and the m. p. was 132 – 135 ℃.

5　Notes

(1) When monitoring the dihydroartemisinin in the reaction progress with TLC, the recommended eluent is petroleum ether: ethyl acetate = 2: 1. However, different thin layers silica gel plate may lead to produce different results. The polarity of the developing solvents should be adjusted according to the initial thin layer results. Artesunate exhibits great polarity and would cause serious tailing on the layer, and therefore, this mobile phase is mainly used to observe the residue of dihydroartemisinin.

(2) During the extraction procedure in this experiment, the concentration of H$_2$SO$_4$ solution for extraction should not be excessive.

(3) If the solid obtained is too sticky, resting the mixture for some time, and stirring with a glass rod could help with the solid transformation.

6　Questions

(1) How to remove the dihydroartemisinin residue in the mixture by extraction in the posttreatment post-processing?

(2) Triethylamine is used as the base in this experiment. Is it appropriate to use NaOH to replace triethylamine?

(3) Please discuss what the most significant difference between dihydroartemisinin and artesunate is in the IR and ^{1}H-NMR spectra.

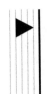

实验九 青蒿素类化合物油水分配系数的测定（薄层色谱法）

一、实验目的

（1）了解油水分配系数在药物设计中的意义。
（2）掌握油水分配系数测定的常用方法和原理。

二、实验原理

油水分配系数 P 是药物设计中一个重要的理化参数，其定义为药物在生物相和水相中的浓度之比。

$$P = C_{生物相}/C_{水相}$$

在药物设计中，P 值主要是用于表征化合物透过脂质双分子层构成的生物膜能力的重要参数。在药物化学家 Christopher A. Lipinski 1997 年归纳的"成药五规则"（Rule of Five）中，其中一条就是化合物的 Log $P \leqslant 5$。一般来说，药物要有一个较为合适的油水分配系数才能在人体内顺利完成溶解、吸收、转运、分布，并最终透过细胞膜进入细胞内与靶点作用从而产生药效，过高或过低的油水分配系数都不利于这一过程。因此，油水分配系数对于合理的药物设计非常重要。由于不同化合物的油水分配系数差距很大，因此我们常用 Log P 值来表示。另外，由于难以直接在生物相中测试 P 值，因此，常用有机相和水相来模拟，最常用的有正辛醇/水相体系。

常用的油水分配系数的测定方法有很多，如摇瓶法、反相高效液相色谱法和反相薄层色谱法等。

摇瓶法是测定油水分配系数的传统方法，但准确性和精密度较差，而且实验操作烦琐和费时，需要使用大量纯化合物。

反相高效液相色谱法利用反相填料的键合非极性疏水表面和极性的流动相来模拟生物膜/水相体系，该方法可以同时进行多种化合物的油水分配系数测定，但测定的准确性取决于建立线性关系的标准化合物。当测定一些结构复杂或不常见的化合物时，往往难以找到建立线性关系的标准化合物。

反相薄层色谱法和高效液相色谱法类似，但是具有使用溶剂量少、分析时间较短和不需要依赖仪器等优点[1-2]。

三、实验方法

（一）设备与材料

展开槽：垂直展开槽。

反相薄层板：RP$_{18}$F$_{254}$（1.05559.0001，Merck，Germany），铝板切成 5 cm×4 cm 备用。

展开体系：甲醇/水。

测试化合物：青蒿素，双氢青蒿素，蒿甲醚，青蒿琥酯。测试化合物配成 3 mg/mL 甲醇储备液。

标准化合物：乙酰苯胺，蒽，对溴苯乙酮和二苯甲酮。标准物质配成 1 mg/mL 甲醇储备液（蒽较难溶于甲醇，可用氯仿：甲醇=1∶1 进行溶解）。

显色方法：碘熏，硫酸-香草醛溶液（配制方法：将 15 g 香草醛溶于 250 mL 无水乙醇，随后向其中慢慢滴入 2.5 mL 的浓 H$_2$SO$_4$）。

（二）操作步骤

（1）展开剂的配制：甲醇/水（%，v/v）浓度范围为 40%～60% 时，每个梯度间隔 10%；浓度范围为 60%～95% 时，每个梯度间隔 5%（每个化合物预试）（表 9-1）。

表 9-1　展开剂的配制

化合物	展开剂：甲醇/水（%，v/v）									
	40%	50%	60%	65%	70%	75%	80%	85%	90%	95%
乙酰苯胺	√	√	√		√		√		√	
对溴苯乙酮				√	√	√	√	√	√	√
二苯甲酮				√	√	√	√	√	√	√
蒽					√	√	√	√	√	√
青蒿素				√	√	√	√	√	√	√
双氢青蒿素				√	√	√	√	√	√	√
蒿甲醚				√	√	√	√	√	√	√
青蒿琥酯				√	√	√	√	√	√	√

（2）往展开槽加入展开剂预饱和 10 min。

（3）化合物在纯水溶剂条件下保留常数 R_{M0} 的测定：将薄层板切开成 5 cm×4 cm，在距离底端 0.7 cm 位置画一条起始线，样品溶液点在起始线上，每个样品点 3 个点。将薄层板放入预饱和的展开槽中展开至溶剂前沿距顶部边沿 0.5 cm 左右，停止展开，在溶剂前沿位置画一条线，薄层干燥后，用碘熏或者喷硫酸 – 香草醛溶液，计算各个点的比移值 R_f 和某个化合物在某个展开剂梯度下的平均 R_f 值。再根据公式计算化合物在该展开条件下的保留常数 R_M。

$$R_M = Log[(1 - R_f)/R_f] = Log[(1/R_f) - 1]$$

将不同展开梯度下该物质的不同的 R_M 进行线性回归，外推计算出当有机溶剂浓度为 0% 时，化合物在纯水相和固定相中的保留常数 R_{M0}。

$$R_M = R_{M0} + bC$$

其中，C 代表甲醇的浓度（%，v/v）；R_{M0} 代表该直线在 Y 轴上的截距；b 为斜率。

（4）标准物质的标准曲线的制备：按上述化合物 R_{M0} 测试方法测试 4 个标准物质（乙酰苯胺、对溴苯乙酮、二苯甲酮和蒽）的 R_{M0}，将文献采用高效液相色谱法测得的这 4 个标准物质的 $Log P_{lit}$ 值与测试的 R_{M0} 值进行线性回归，也就是在本实验方法和环境条件下测得的 R_M 值与文献实测值之间建立对应关系。得到 k，m 和回归相关系数 r。

$$Log P_{lit} = k R_{M0} + m$$

（5）计算 $Log P_{TLC}$：将标准物质和待测化合物的 R_{M0} 值代入上述回归公式中，可以计算出各标准物质及待测化合物在本次实验环境中测得的 $Log P_{TLC}$（表 9 – 2，表 9 – 3）。

表 9 – 2　标准物质的 R_{M0} 和 $Log P_{TLC}$ 计算结果汇总

化合物	$Log P_{lit}$	R_{M0}	b	r	$Log P_{TLC}$
乙酰苯胺	1.21				
对溴苯乙酮	2.43				
二苯甲酮	3.18				
蒽	4.45				

注：b 是斜率，$R_M = R_{M0} + bC$，r 是该方程线性回归的相关系数。

表 9 – 3　待测化合物的 R_{M0} 和 $Log P_{TLC}$ 计算结果汇总

化合物	R_{M0}	b	r	$Log P_{TLC}$
青蒿素				
双氢青蒿素				
蒿甲醚				
青蒿琥酯				

注：b 是斜率，$R_M = R_{M0} + bC$，r 是该方程线性回归的相关系数。

（6）将获得的青蒿素衍生物的 Log P_{TLC} 值与表9－4中文献报道的值进行对比。

表9－4　青蒿素衍生物的 Log P_{TLC} 值与文献报道的值的对比

化合物	Log P_{lit}	溶解度/（mg·L^{-1}）
青蒿素	2.27[4]	
青蒿素	2.94[8]	63
双氢青蒿素（α）	1.58[7]	
双氢青蒿素（β）	2.19[7]	
蒿甲醚（pH）	2.2（水），1.6（5），1.5（6.8），2.6（7.4），2.2（8.0）[5]	
蒿甲醚（α）	2.05[7]	
蒿甲醚（β）	2.86[7]	
蒿甲醚	3.98[8]	117
青蒿琥酯	2.4（水），3.36（4），2.84（5），2.33（5.8），2.21（6.8），2.25（7.4），2.23（8）[6]	
青蒿琥酯	2.77[8]	565

（7）实验拓展：化合物的理论油水分配系数，可以在 http：//www. vcclab. org/lab/alogps/进行计算得到[3]，将得到的计算值与实测值对比，并进行线性回归，根据每个计算模型的回归方程，可评估出哪个计算模型在青蒿素衍生物的油水分配系数的计算和预测中具有更高的精度（表9－5，表9－6）。

表9－5　青蒿素衍生物的油水分配系数的计算值

化合物	ALOGPs	AClogP	miLogP	ALOGP	MLOGP	XLOGP2	XLOGP3
青蒿素							
双氢青蒿素							
蒿甲醚							
青蒿琥酯							

表9－6　青蒿素衍生物不同计算方法理论值对实测值的回归分析

软件	b	C	r	SD
ALOGPs				
AClogP				

续表 9 – 6

软件	b	C	r	SD
miLogP				
ALOGP				
MLOGP				
XLOGP2				
XLOGP3				

注：b 是斜率，$\log P_{TLC} = b \log P_{calc} + C$，r 是该方程线性回归的相关系数。

四、附注

（1）通过预筛选的方法确定化合物的溶剂选择和溶剂配比范围，取有机溶剂/水从 5%～95%，每间隔 15% 设一个浓度点，一般合适的溶剂应该在合适的 R_f 值范围内有较大的溶剂配比范围。

（2）加入的展开剂的量不能没过样品起始线。

（3）碘熏之前先把薄层板上的有机溶剂吹干；采用硫酸 – 香草醛溶液显色，喷板后须在 110 ℃ 烘箱（或热枪）中干燥显色。标准物质可以在紫外检测器 254 nm 和碘熏两种途径观察到明显的样品点，但青蒿素衍生物在碘熏下显色灵敏度很低，在硫酸 – 香草醛溶液中显色灵敏度大幅度提高。

（4）用铅笔把化合物的点和起止线标注好后，建议用 TLC Chemistry 或者 TLC to flash&prep App 来计算 R_f 值。

五、思考题

（1）根据测得的青蒿素衍生物的 Log P 值，试解释为何蒿甲醚的活性要好于青蒿素？

（2）本次试验的青蒿琥酯是采用甲醇/水体系进行测量，如果将水换成酸性或碱性的缓冲溶液，那么它的 Log P 值将如何变化？

（3）对比测得的青蒿素衍生物的 Log P 值，发现青蒿琥酯与青蒿素及双氢青蒿素之间差别不大，但为何青蒿琥酯可以做成注射剂，用于脑型疟及各种危重疟疾的抢救？

Experiment 9 Determining the Oil-Water Partition Coefficient of Artemisinin Derivatives (Thin Layer Chromatography)

1 Learning Objectives

(1) To understand what the oil-water partition coefficient is in the drug design.

(2) To master the experimental method and principles of determining the oil-water partition coefficient.

2 Experimental Principle

The oil-water partition coefficient, P, is an important physicochemical parameter in drug design. It is defined as the concentration ratio of drugs in the biological phase and aquatic phase as follows:

$$P = C_{\text{biological phases}}/C_{\text{aquatic phases}}$$

In drug design, the P value is an important parameter defining the ability of chemical compounds to penetrate through biological membranes composed of lipid bilayers. Christopher A. Lipinski, a medicinal chemist, summarized the "Rules of Five" in 1997. One of the principles is that the Log P of the oil-water partition coefficient should not be greater than 5. In general, a drug must exhibit a suitable oil-water partition coefficient to achieve dissolution, absorption, transport, and distribution in the body. Penetrate the cell membranes to enter the cells and interact with targets, and produce drug effects. Neither excessively high nor excessively low partition coefficients are conducive to this process. Therefore, the oil-water partition coefficient is very important for designing drugs appropriately. Since the oil-water partition coefficient of different compounds varies widely, Log P value is often used to represent the coefficient. Furthermore, since it is difficult to directly determine the P value in the biological phase, the organic phase and water phase are often used for simulation, and the most commonly used system is the n-octanol/water phase.

There are many methods for determining the oil-water partition coefficient, such as the shake-flask method, reversed phase high performance liquid chromatography and reversed phase thin layer chromatography.

The shake flask method is a traditional method for determining the oil-water partition coefficient. However, this method exhibits poor accuracy and precision, and the experimental operation is cumbersome and time-consuming, and many pure compounds are needed.

Reversed phase high performance liquid chromatography utilizes the bonded nonpolar hydrophobic surface of the reversed phase packing and polar mobile phase to simulate the biofilm/water phase system. This method can simultaneously determine the oil-water partition coefficients of various compounds. The accuracy depends on the standard compounds, which are used to establish a linear relationship. However, when measuring some compounds with complex or uncommon structures, it is difficult to find standard compounds that establish a linear relationship.

Reversed phase thin layer chromatography is similar to high performance liquid chromatography but exhibits several advantages, i. e. less solvent consumption, shorter analyzing time, and no instrumental requirement[1-2].

3 Experimental Procedure

3.1 Equipment and materials

Developing tank: vertical tank.

Reverse phase thin layer plate: $RP_{18}F_{254}$ (1. 05559. 0001, Merck, Germany) , aluminum sheet cut into 5 cm ×4 cm.

Developing solvent system: methanol/water.

Tested compounds: artemisinin, dihydroartemisinin, artemether, artesunate; tested compounds were respectively made into 3 mg/mL methanol stock solutions.

Standard compounds: acetanilide, anthracene, 4-bromoacetophenone and benzophenone; the standard compounds were made into a 1 mg/mL methanol stock solution (anthracene is difficult to dissolve in methanol and can be dissolved in chloroform : methanol = 1 : 1)

Color development method: iodine fumigation, sulfuric-acid-vanillin solution (preparation method: dissolve 15 g of vanillin into 250 mL of absolute ethanol, and then add 2. 5 mL of concentrated H_2SO_4 into the solution) .

3.2 Operation procedures

(1) Preparing the developing solvent: when the concentration range of methanol/water (% , v/v) is 40% to 60% , the interval of each gradient is 10% ; when the concentration of methanol/water (% , v/v) is 60% to 90% , the interval of each gradient is 5% (pretest for each compound) (Table 9 – 1) .

Table 9 –1   The preparation of the developing solvent

Compound	Developing solvent: methanol/water (% , v/v)									
	40%	50%	60%	65%	70%	75%	80%	85%	90%	95%
Acetanilide	√	√	√		√		√		√	
4-Bromoacetophenone				√	√	√	√	√	√	√
Benzophenone				√	√	√	√	√	√	√
Anthracene						√	√	√	√	√
Artemisinin				√	√	√	√	√	√	√

Table 9 – 1 (Continued)

Compound	Developing solvent: methanol/water (%, v/v)									
	40%	50%	60%	65%	70%	75%	80%	85%	90%	95%
Dihydroartemisinin				√	√	√	√	√	√	√
Artemether				√	√	√	√	√	√	√
Artesunate				√	√	√	√	√	√	√

(2) Add the developing solvent to the developing tank for presaturation for 10 min.

(3) Determination of R_{M0} of the compounds: cut the thin layer plate into 5 cm × 4 cm pieces, draw a line at a distance of 0.7 cm from the bottom end, and apply the spots of the sample on the starting line with three spots for each sample. Place the plate in the presaturated developing tank, and stop expansion when the solvent front is approximately 0.5 cm away from the tank top. Draw a line at the solvent front. After the plate is dried, fumigate the plate with iodine or spray the sulfuric-acid-vanillin solution on the plate . Calculate the R_f value of each spot and the average R_f value of each compound under a certain developing solvent gradient. Then, calculate the retention constants (R_M) of the compound under this expansion condition according to the following equation:

$$R_M = Log [(1 - R_f)/R_f] = Log [(1/R_f) - 1]$$

The different values of R_M of the compound under different developing solvent gradients are analyzed by linear regression, and calculate the R_{M0} parameter by extrapolating methanol concentration to zero according to the equation:

$$R_M = R_{M0} + bC$$

where C represents the concentration of methanol (%, v/v); R_{M0} represents the intercept of the line on the Y axis; b represents the slope of the equation.

(4) Drawing the standard curve for the standard compounds: determine the R_{M0} of the standard compounds following the method above (acetanilide, 4-bromoacetophenone, benzophenone and anthracene). Perform linear regression between the oil-water distribution coefficients (Log P_{lit}) of the four standard compounds determined by HPLC in the literature and the determined R_{M0} values; that is, establish a corresponding relationship between the R_M measured in this experimental method and environmental conditions and the experimental data in the literature. Calculate the k value and m value and the regression correlation coefficient r.

$$Log P_{lit} = k R_{M0} + m$$

(5) Calculation of the oil-water partition coefficient (Log P_{TLC}): substitute the R_{M0} values of the standard compounds and the compounds to be tested into the above regression formula, and calculate the Log P_{TLC} of each standard compounds and the compounds to be

tested in this experimental environment (Table 9 – 2, Table 9 – 3).

Table 9 – 2　Summary of results for the R_{mo} and Log P_{TLC} of the standard compounds

Compound	Log P_{lit}	R_{MO}	b	r	Log P_{TLC}
Acetanilide	1. 21				
4 – Bromoacetophenone	2. 43				
Benzophenone	3. 18				
Anthracene	4. 45				

Notes: b represents the slope, $R_M = R_{MO} + bC$; r represents the correlation coefficient.

Table 9 – 3　Summary of the calculations for the R_{mo} and Log P_{TLC} of the tested compounds

Compound	R_{MO}	b	r	Log P_{TLC}
Artemisinin				
Dihydroartemisinin				
Artemether				
Artesunate				

Notes: b represents the slope, $R_M = R_{MO} + bC$; r represents the correlation coefficient.

(6) The Log P_{TLC} values of the obtained artemisinin derivatives were compared with the values reported in the literature (Table 9 – 4).

Table 9 – 4　Comparison of log P_{TLC} values of artemisinin derivatives with values reports in the literature

Compound	Log P_{lit}	Solubility/($mg \cdot L^{-1}$)
Artemisinin	2. 27[4]	
Artemisinin	2. 94[8]	63
Dihydroartemisinin (α)	1. 58[7]	
Dihydroartemisinin (β)	2. 19[7]	
Artemether (pH)	2. 2 (water), 1. 6 (5), 1. 5 (6. 8), 2. 6 (7. 4), 2. 2 (8. 0)[5]	
Artemether (α)	2. 05[7]	
Artemether (β)	2. 86[7]	
Artemether	3. 98[8]	117
Artesunate	2. 4 (water), 3. 36 (4), 2. 84 (5), 2. 33 (5. 8), 2. 21 (6. 8), 2. 25 (7. 4), 2. 23 (8)[6]	
Artesunate	2. 77[8]	565

（7）Experiment extension: the theoretical oil-water partition coefficients of the compounds can be calculated at http://www.vcclab.org/lab/alogps/[3]. The calculated values are compared with the measured values, and the linear regression is performed. By analyzing the regression equation of each computational software, it is possible to determine which computational software has higher accuracy in the calculation and prediction of the oil-water partition coefficient of artemisinin derivatives (Table 9 – 5, Table 9 – 6).

Table 9 –5   Calculated values of the oil-water partition coefficients of the artemisinin derivatives

Compound	ALOGPs	AClogP	miLogP	ALOGP	MLOGP	XLOGP2	XLOGP3
Artemisinin							
Dihydroartemisinin							
Artemether							
Artesunate							

Table 9 –6   Regression analysis of the computational procedures versus experimental data

Software	b	C	r	SD
ALOGPs				
AClogP				
miLogP				
ALOGP				
MLOGP				
XLOGP2				
XLOGP3				

Notes: b represents the slope, $\log P_{TLC} = b \log P_{calc} + C$, C represents intercepts, r represents the correlation coefficient.

4   Notes

（1）The prescreening method can be used to select the solvent for the compounds and determine the solvent ratio. The concentration range of the organic solvent/water is 5% to 95%, with the concentration point every 15% interval. Generally, suitable solvent should exhibit a large range of solvent ratios within the appropriate R_f.

（2）Never allow the starting lines immersed by the developing solvent.

（3）Dry the organic solvent on the thin layer plate before performing iodine fumigation. Alternatively, dry the thin layer plate in a 110 ℃ oven (or with a heat gun) for color development after spraying the plate with the sulfuric-acid-vanillin solution. The spots of standard compounds can be easily observed under a 254 nm UV detector or iodine fumigation. The chromogenic sensitivity of artemisinin derivatives is low under iodine fumigation, but it can be greatly improved with the sulfuric-acid-vanillin solution.

(4) After marking the sample spots, the starting lines and ending lines with pencils, it is recommended to use TLC Chemistry or TLC to flash&prep App to calculate R_f value.

5　Questions

(1) Based on the Log P values for the tested artemisinin derivatives, explain why the activity of artemether is better than that of artemisinin.

(2) The artesunate in this experiment is measured in a methanol/water system. If one replaces water with an acidic or basic buffer solution, how will the Log P value change?

(3) Regarding the Log P values for the tested artemisinin derivatives, there is little difference between artesunate, artemisinin and dihydroartemisinin. However, why can artesunate be utilized in injections to rescue cerebral malaria or other critical malaria?

References

[1] BOBER K, BEBENEK E, BORYCZK S. Application of TLC for evaluation of the lipophilicity of newly synthetized esters: betulin derivatives[J]. Journal of analytical methods in chemistry, 2019, 1297659.

[2] PETROVIC S M, ONCARE L, KOLAROV L et al. Correlation between retention and 1-octanol-water partition coefficients of some estrane derivatives in reversed-phase thin-layer chromatography[J]. Journal of chromatographic science, 2002, 40 (10), 569 – 574.

[3] TETKO I V, GASTEIGER J, TODESCHINI R, et al. Virtual computational chemistry laboratory-design and description[J]. Journal of computer-aided molecular design, 2005, 19 (6): 453 – 63.

[4] 王振华, 梁家龙, 曾令清, 等. HPLC-ECD 法测定青蒿素溶解度及油水分配系数[J]. 中药新药与临床药理, 2014, 25 (3): 352 – 356.

[5] 王晓蕾, 孙艺丹, 王锐利, 等. 蒿甲醚在不同介质中的平衡溶解度及表观油水分配系数的测定[J]. 药物评价研究, 2013, 36 (2): 114 – 118.

[6] 沈硕, 刘淑芝, 杜茂波, 等. 青蒿琥酯平衡溶解度和表观油水分配系数的测定[J]. 中国实验方剂学杂志, 2013, 19 (19): 9 – 12.

[7] 吴吉安, 嵇汝运. 青蒿素衍生物的油水分配系数与抗疟活性之间的 Hansch 分析[J]. 中国药理学报, 1982, 3 (1): 55 – 60.

[8] 郭宗儒. 青蒿素类抗疟药的研制[J]. 药学学报, 2016, 51 (1): 157 – 164.

实验十 烷胺基甲酸芳酯的合成、乙酰胆碱酯酶 抑制活性测试及构效关系分析

一、实验目的

（1）掌握两种不同的酯化反应方法。
（2）掌握硅胶柱层析分离纯化技术。
（3）了解乙酰胆碱酯酶（acetylcholinesterase，AChE）活性筛选技术的原理和方法。
（4）了解常用构效关系分析的手段和原理。

二、实验原理和实验方法

（一）烷胺基甲酸芳酯的合成

1. 实验原理

方法一：如图 10-1 所示。

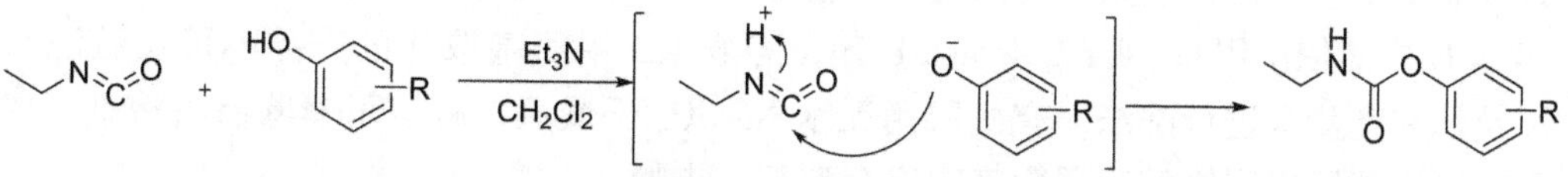

图 10-1 烷胺基甲酸芳酯的合成（方法一）

方法二：如图 10-2 所示。

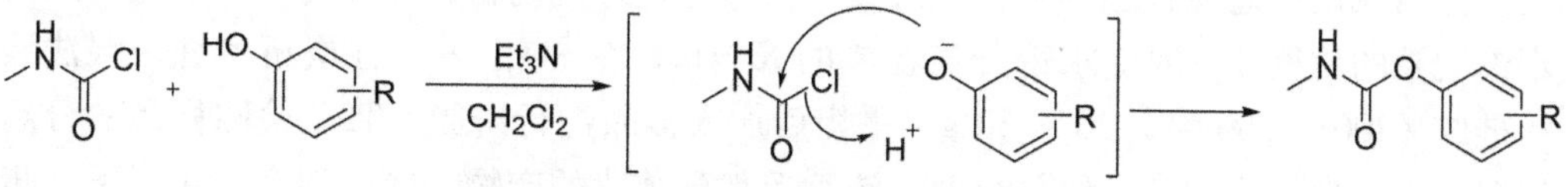

图 10-2 烷胺基甲酸芳酯的合成（方法二）

2. 实验方法

（1）实验试剂：实验用试剂的规格和用量见表 10-1。

表 10 - 1　实验试剂规格和用量

试剂	规格	用量 （重量和体积）	物质的量/ mmol	摩尔比	安全信息
异氰酸乙酯（方法一）	分析纯	—	9	1.5	
甲胺基甲酰氯（方法二）	分析纯	—			
酚	分析纯	—	6	1	
三乙胺	分析纯	—	12	2	
二氯甲烷	分析纯	35 mL（方法一） 40 mL（方法二）			

注：其他试剂包括乙酸乙酯、无水 $CaCl_2$、无水 Na_2SO_4、饱和食盐水、4 mol/L HCl 溶液。

（2）操作步骤。

A. 方法一：称量 6 mmol 酚置于 50 mL 反应瓶，加入 5 mL 二氯甲烷和 12 mmol 三乙胺，混匀后加入 9 mmol 异氰酸乙酯，加上干燥管，室温下搅拌反应，通过 TLC 监测反应进程，至原料酚消失（一般需 0.5～1.0 h）。反应结束后，加入 30 mL 的二氯甲烷，反应液依次用水、4 mL 4 mol/L HCl 溶液（二甲氨基取代的产品不可用酸洗），以及饱和食盐水进行洗涤，分出有机层用无水 Na_2SO_4 干燥后，减压下蒸除有机溶剂，残留物可以放置在同样的容器中密闭保存到下一步骤。

B. 方法二：称量 6 mmol 酚置于 50 mL 反应瓶，加入 10 mL 二氯甲烷和 12 mmol 三乙胺，混匀后加入 9 mmol 甲胺基甲酰氯，加上干燥管，室温下搅拌反应，通过 TLC 监测反应进程，至原料酚消失（一般需 1～2 h）。反应结束后，加入二氯甲烷 30 mL，反应液依次用水、4 mL 4 mol/L HCl 溶液（二甲氨基取代的产品不可用酸洗），以及饱和食盐水进行洗涤，有机层用无水 Na_2SO_4 干燥后，减压下蒸除有机溶剂，残留物可以放置在同样的容器中密闭保存到下一步骤。

（二）烷胺基甲酸芳酯的纯化

将上一步得到的粗品溶于少量的二氯甲烷中，置于培养皿中，加入 5 g 左右的硅胶，在通风橱中边搅拌边挥发至硅胶无结块并呈良好流动状，拌样完毕。通过薄层确定洗脱液的比例（一般要求待分离物质的 $R_f = 0.3$ 左右）。另取柱层析空柱，湿法装入硅胶（200～300 目）20～30 g，平衡后加入样品进行洗脱，TLC 检测样品的分离情况，对分离纯化的产品组分合并，浓缩后得到纯化的产物，密闭保存，用于下一步的分析测试。

化合物的结构确证：对纯化后的产品进行熔点、IR 和 ^{1}H-NMR 数据的收集，并对其结构进行解析。

（三）化合物对乙酰胆碱酯酶抑制活性测试

1. 实验原理

乙酰胆碱酯酶抑制剂的活性测试方法基于 Ellman 法，它是一种利用紫外光谱进行测定的方法。其原理如下：当乙酰胆碱酯酶水解底物硫代乙酰胆碱后，会产生硫代胆碱。它与 5, 5′ – 二硫代双（2 – 硝基苯甲酸）［5, 5′-dithiobis- （2-nitrobenzoic acid），DTNB］反应产生黄色的 5 – 巯基 – 2 – 硝基苯甲酸，并在 412 nm 处有紫外吸收，5 – 巯基 – 2 – 硝基苯甲酸的生成速率与酶的活性呈正相关。其反应过程如图 10 – 3 所示：

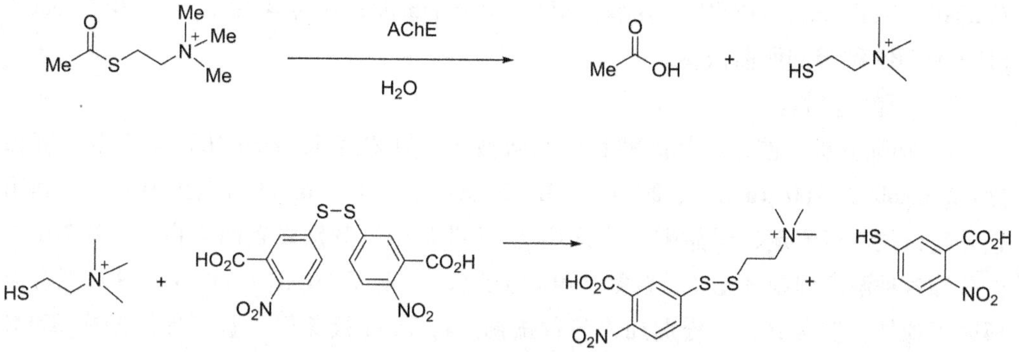

图 10 – 3　乙酰胆碱酯酶抑制剂活性测试原理

进行活性测试时，小分子与乙酰胆碱酯酶处于体系中，加入底物后，小分子与底物共同竞争酶的催化位点。当小分子对酶有抑制活性时，会使酶对底物的水解减少，产生黄色的 5 – 巯基 – 2 – 硝基苯甲酸也减少，因此在 412 nm 处测定的紫外吸收值就会比阴性对照小。紫外吸收值越低，表明小分子的抑制活性越好。

IC_{50} 是用来表征活性小分子对酶抑制活性的一种指标，是指使酶的活性降为未加任何物质时活性的一半时所加抑制剂的浓度。因此，活性小分子的 IC_{50} 越小，其对酶的抑制活性越高。酶活力可用一定条件下酶催化某一化学反应的反应速率表示，反应速率越快，酶的活力越高；反应速率越慢，酶的活力越低。在实验中，通过测定酶催化化学反应的速率可以得到酶的活力，而这种反应速率可用单位时间内底物的减少量或产物的生成量表示。

2. 乙酰胆碱酯酶抑制活性的测试方法

（1）缓冲溶液的配制方法。

A. 0.1 mol/L pH 8.0 磷酸盐缓冲溶液（phosphate butter saline，PBS）：取 1.0 mol/L K_2HPO_4 水溶液 94 mL 和 1.0 mol/L KH_2PO_4 的水溶液 6 mL，混匀，用去离子水稀释，调节溶液 pH 至 8.0，定容至 1 000 mL，保存于 4 ℃备用。

B. 乙酰胆碱酯酶溶液（现用现配）：乙酰胆碱酯酶浓溶液（约2.5 U/μL）用0.1 mol/L pH 8.0 PBS 稀释为0.5～2 U/mL，以事先测定的活性确定稀释倍数。

C. 0.01 mol/L 硫代乙酰胆碱（acetylthiocholine，ATC）溶液：称取31.6 mg 硫代乙酰胆碱用0.1 mol/L pH 8.0 PBS 15.0 mL 溶解，4 ℃遮光保存。

D. 0.01 mol/L DTNB 溶液：称取59.4 mg DTNB 用0.1 mol/L pH 8.0 PBS 15.0 mL 溶解，4 ℃遮光保存，用棕色 EP 管分装。

E. ATC + DTNB 混合液：将上述配好的 ATC 与 DTNB 溶液以1∶1 的比例混合，现配现用。

F. 50.0 mmol/L 样品溶液：称取一定量各种待分析样品用适量二甲基亚砜（dimethyl sulfoxide，DMSO）溶解，配成 50.0 mmol/L 样品溶液，再用 0.1 mol/L pH 8.0 PBS 稀释到所需浓度。

（2）操作步骤。

A. 初筛分析：首先用 PBS 稀释样品溶液（初始浓度 50 mmol/L）至 5 个浓度梯度：2 mmol/L、200 μmol/L、20 μmol/L，2 μmol/L 和 0.2 μmol/L（图 10 - 4）。利用紫外酶标仪进行测定，样品配制在透明的 96 孔板中。分别设置酶空白孔、DTNB 空白孔和各种浓度抑制剂孔（设置复孔可减少误差），除了 DTNB + ATC（1∶1）混合液暂时不加外，按表 10 - 2 分别加入各种试剂。将 96 孔板盖好，置于保温箱中 37 ℃孵育 10 min。孵育完后，加入 DTNB + ATC（1∶1）混合液，立即用酶标仪进行检测。酶标仪的设置为：自动振荡 10 s，读取每个样品孔在 412 nm 处的紫外吸收曲线，即酶的催化曲线，收集 3 min 内的数据，每个数据点间隔时间 15 s。

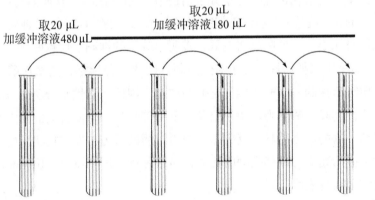

图 10 - 4 指定浓度的样品的稀释方法（10 倍稀释）

表 10 - 2　初筛分析中各加样孔的样品加入种类和加样量

试剂加样量	抑制剂					酶空白	DTNB空白	对照
	2 000 μmol/L	200 μmol/L	20 μmol/L	2 μmol/L	0.2 μmol/L			
缓冲液/μL	20	20	20	20	20	100	90	80
抑制剂/μL	60	60	60	60	60	0	0	0
DTNB/μL	0	0	0	0	0	0	10	0
AChE/μL	20	20	20	20	20	20	20	20
DTNB + ATC	20	20	20	20	20	0	0	20
总体积/μL	120	120	120	120	120	120	120	120
终浓度/($\mu mol/L^{-1}$)	1 000	100	10	1	0.1			

注：DTNB + ATC 的样品用多道移液枪加入。缓冲液、抑制剂、DTNB 和 AChE 于孵育前加入，DTNB + ATC 于测量前加入。

B. IC_{50} 测试：根据上述初筛结果，确定化合物抑制活性的大致范围，以倍半稀释的方法设置一系列化合物的浓度（图 10 - 5），使其覆盖化合物抑制活性所在的范围，再按表 10 - 3 的试剂和剂量配制测试液（可根据需要增减测试范围和测试点数量），再按初筛方法进行测试。

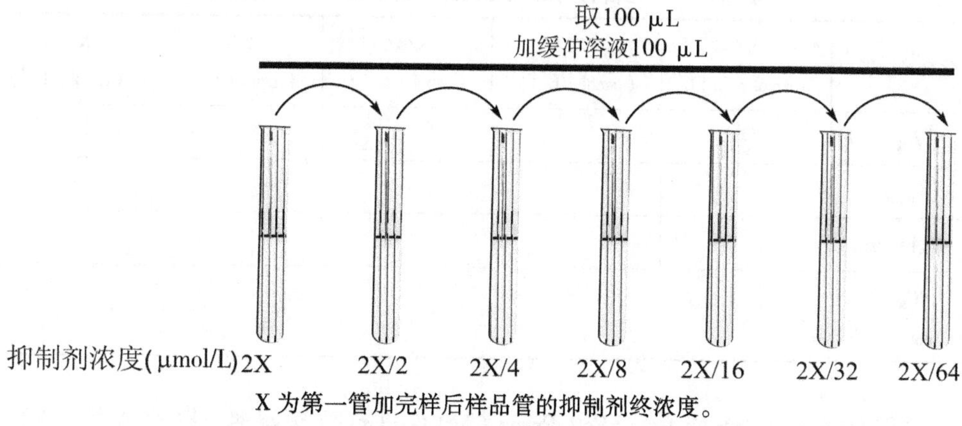

取 100 μL
加缓冲溶液 100 μL

抑制剂浓度(μmol/L) 2X　　2X/2　　2X/4　　2X/8　　2X/16　　2X/32　　2X/64

X 为第一管加完样后样品管的抑制剂终浓度。

图 10 - 5　指定浓度的样品的稀释方法（倍半稀释）

表 10 - 3　IC_{50} 分析中各加样孔的样品加入试剂种类和加样量

试剂加样量	抑制剂							酶空白	DTNB空白	对照
	2 X μmol/L	2 X/2 μmol/L	2 X/4 μmol/L	2 X/8 μmol/L	2 X/16 μmol/L	2 X/32 μmol/L	2 X/64 μmol/L			
缓冲液/μL	20	20	20	20	20	20	20	100	90	80
抑制剂/μL	60	60	60	60	60	60	60	0	0	0
DTNB/μL	0	0	0	0	0	0	0	0	10	0

续表 10 – 3

试剂加样量	抑制剂							酶空白	DTNB空白	对照
	2 X μmol/L	2 X/2 μmol/L	2 X/4 μmol/L	2 X/8 μmol/L	2 X/16 μmol/L	2 X/32 μmol/L	2 X/64 μmol/L			
AChE/μL	20	20	20	20	20	20	20	20	20	20
DTNB + ATC	20	20	20	20	20	20	20	0	0	20
总体积/μL	120	120	120	120	120	120	120	120	120	120
终浓度/ (μmol·L^{-1})	X	X/2	X/4	X/8	X/16	X/32	X/64			

注：DTNB + ATC 的样品用多道移液枪加入，X 为第一管加完样品管的抑制剂终浓度。DTNB + ATC 的样品用多道移液枪加入。缓冲液、抑制剂、DTNB 和 ACHE 于孵育前加入，DTNB + ATC 于测量前加入。

C. 数据处理：将 DTNB 空白作为实验本底，以酶对照和小分子抑制剂的数据分别减去 DTNB 空白所得到的值对时间作图，将每个系列的点进行线性拟合，得到方程 $y = Kx + B$，斜率 K 即代表酶的相对活性（表 10 – 4）。小分子抑制剂的抑制活性可以通过以下公式计算：

$$抑制率（\%）= （1 - K_{抑制剂}/K_{酶}）\times 100\%$$

表 10 –4   化合物对乙酰胆碱酯酶抑制活性 IC$_{50}$ 的计算

化合物浓度	X/ (μmol·L^{-1})	X/2/ (μmol·L^{-1})	X/4/ (μmol·L^{-1})	X/8/ (μmol·L^{-1})	X/16/ (μmol·L^{-1})
$K_{酶}$					
$K_{抑制剂}$					
抑制率/%					
IC_{50}/ (μmol·L^{-1})					

采用 Origin、SPSS 或 GraphPad Prism 等软件进行数据处理，以抑制率（%）对 $LogC_{抑制剂}$ 做散点图，进行非线性回归（nonlinear regression）拟合，求出 IC$_{50}$ 值。将个人及班级其他同学的测试数据汇总入表 10 – 5（相同化合物多组测试数据要对结果进行平均化）。

表 10 −5　实验系列化合物对乙酰胆碱酯酶抑制活性 IC_{50} 结果汇总

| | $R_1 = -CH_3$ | | $R_1 = -C_2H_5$ | |
R_2	实测 $IC_{50}/$ ($\mu mol \cdot L^{-1}$)	文献 $IC_{50}/$ ($\mu mol \cdot L^{-1}$)	实测 $IC_{50}/$ ($\mu mol \cdot L^{-1}$)	文献 $IC_{50}/$ ($\mu mol \cdot L^{-1}$)
− H		200		
2 − Br		2.2		
2 − i − Pr		6.0		
3 − F		85		
3 − Cl		50		
3 − Br		13		
3 − I		7.0		
3 − CH₃		14		
3 − C₂H₅		4.8		
3 − i − Pr		0.34		
3 − OCH₃		22		
3 − i − OPr		9.2		
3 − N (CH₃)₂		8		
4 − Br		88		
4 − CH₃		—		
4 − i − Pr		70		
4 − OCH₃		80		
Ar = − 1 − 萘基		0.9		
Ar = -2 − 萘基		14		
3,5 − 二甲基		6.0		

（四）构效关系分析

1. 实验原理

定量构效关系（quantitative structure-activity relationship，QSAR）指研究一组化合物的生物活性与结构特征之间的相互关系，结构特征以理化参数、分子拓扑参数、量子化学指数和结构碎片指数来表示，用数理统计的方法进行数据回归分析，并以数学模型表达和概括出量变规律。由于数学模型大多由化合物的二维结构得出，因此将这类定量构效关系研究定义为2D-QSAR。

Hansch-Fujita 分析是 2D-QSAR 中最常用的构效关系分析方法，其依据是药物在体内的运转和与受体的相互作用为药物分子与生物大分子之间的物理和化学作用。药物从给药部位到作用靶点，需要经过若干生物膜及一定数量的脂 - 水界面，因此药物的转运与药物的脂水分配系数有关，而药物到达靶点浓度的高低影响药物作用的强度。药物通过共价键、离子键、离子 - 偶极键、氢键、疏水键、螯合作用、范德瓦耳斯力等与靶点相互作用产生生物活性，这些作用又与药物分子的化学结构、电子效应、空间效应等相关。Hansch 由此提出同源物的生物活性与各种取代基的理化参数之间存在相关性，用与自由能相关的参数方程（Hansch 方程）表示：

$$\text{Log } (1/C) = -k_1\pi^2 + k_2\pi + k_3\sigma + k_4 MR + k_5$$

式中，C 为化合物产生对应生物效应时的摩尔浓度；π，σ 和 MR 分别为疏水性参数、电性参数和立体参数（表 10 - 6）；k_1、k_2、k_3 和 k_4 分别代表各项因素贡献大小的权重系数，与化合物及测定条件有关。这些系数用最小二乘法，经多元回归分析求出。

表 10 - 6　芳环上取代基的代表性参数

- R	π	σ_m	MR
H	0.00	0.00	1.03
F	0.14	0.34	0.92
Cl	0.71	0.37	6.03
Br	0.86	0.39	8.88
I	1.12	0.35	13.94
CH_3	0.56	-0.07	5.65
CH_2CH_3	1.02	-0.07	10.30
$CH(CH_3)_2$	1.53	-0.07	14.98
$CH_2CH(CH_3)_2$	1.98	-0.10	19.62
OCH_3	-0.02	0.12	7.87
$OCH(CH_3)_2$	0.36	0.10	17.06
$N(CH_3)_2$	0.18	-0.15	15.55

（1）疏水性参数。疏水性参数 π 以药物分子的油水分配系数的对数 Log P 来表征：

$$\pi_x = \text{Log } P_x - \text{Log } P_H$$

式中，Log P_H 为未取代的母体化合物的油水分配系数；Log P_x 为被 X 取代的化合物的油水分配系数。π 为正值时表明该基团亲脂性比氢取代基强，为负值则表明亲水性比氢取代基强。π 值可以从表 10 - 6 中查到，也可以采用色谱参数 R 用于方程计算，或者通过计算软件得到 Log P 值。

（2）电性参数。取代基的电性效应对分子反应性能的影响可以用哈米特（Hammett）方程中的 Hammett 常数（σ 值）来量度。取代基的 σ 值反映了诱导效应和共轭效应之和。在对位时两种效应都有，在间位时只有诱导效应，在邻位时除了以上两种效应外，还有位阻或氢键等引起的邻位效应，此时 σ 须作特殊处理。σ 为正值表示为吸电子基因，为负值表示为给电子基因。σ 值可从表 10 - 6 中查出。

（3）立体参数。有多种参数用于表征取代基的立体因素，这里采用摩尔折射率（molar refractivity，MR）来表征，其定义为：

$$MR = \left[(n^2 - 1)/(n^2 + 2) \right] (MW/d)$$

式中，n 为液体折射率；MW 为分子量；d 为密度；MW/d 为液体的摩尔体积。根据 MR 的加和性质，可以从分子的 MR 求出原子或基团的 MR 值。若方程中 MR 项为负值，即表示空间位阻为重要影响因素；如果为正值，说明由诱导极化产生的色散力为主要影响因素。MR 值可表 10 - 6 中查出。

Hansch 分析只是用于作用机理相同的同源物，即基本结构相同，而取代基不同的系列化合物。在设计化合物时，要对取代基进行选择，使其理化参数有从负到正一定幅度的变化，生物活性数据也要有较大差距（至少一个对数单位以上）。化合物的数目一般至少为理化参数数目的 5 倍，才能保证统计结果的准确性。

Hansch 分析按多元线性回归分析（multiple linear regression，MLR）处理，用最小二乘法求得各因变量的系数，得到回归方程。应用这种方法进行定量构效关系的研究要求方程中各参数间没有或有较小的相关性，各参数在方程式中代表独立变量。

2. 定量构效关系分析

根据 Hansch 方程：

$$Log\ (1/C) = -k_1\pi^2 + k_2\pi + k_3\sigma + k_4\ MR + k_5$$

将表 10 - 6 的各参数和对应的 IC_{50} 值一一列出，填入表 10 - 7。采用 Excel 中的函数 LINEST（［known_y's］，［known_x's］，［const］，［stats］）来进行线性回归。其中，［known_y's］对应 $log\ (1/IC_{50})$ 这一列数值；［known_x's］对应 π^2、π、σ_m 和 MR 这四列数值；［const］取 TRUE 值；［stats］取 TRUE 值。将公式复制到一张空白工作表后，选择以公式单元格开始的一块 5 × 5 的单元格区域。按 F2，然后按 Ctrl + Shift + Enter。如果公式不是以数组公式输入，则返回单个结果值。当作为数组输入时，将返回回归统计值，用该值可识别所需的统计值。回归统计值结果对应的参数意义见表 10 - 8。

表 10 - 7　用于 Hansch 方程分析的各参数资料（仅对位含 R_2 取代基的化合物进行 QSAR 分析）

$3 - R_2$ 取代基	$IC_{50}/$ ($\mu mol \cdot L^{-1}$)	$1/IC_{50}$	$\log (1/IC_{50})$	π^2	π	σ_m	MR
H							
F							
Cl							
Br							
I							
CH_3							
CH_2CH_3							
$CH(CH_3)_2$							
$CH_2CH(CH_3)_2$							
OCH_3							
$OCH(CH_3)_2$							
$N(CH_3)_2$							

表 10 - 8　LINEST 函数输出结果对应的参数意义

k_4	k_3	k_2	k_1	b
se_4	se_3	se_2	se_1	se_b
r^2	Se_y			
F	D_f			
ss_{reg}	Ss_{resid}			

注：k 值对应 Hansch 方程相应的各参数前的系数（Excel 中给出的顺序相反）；se 值是对应系数的标准差；Se_y 为 y 估计值的标准误差；r^2 为判定系数，y 的估计值与实际值之比，样本的相关性越好，r^2 越接近 1；F 为 F 统计，可以判断因变量和自变量之间是否偶尔发生过可观察到的关系；D_f 为自由度，用于在统计表上查找 F 临界值；ss_{reg} 为回归平方和；Ss_{resid} 为残差平方和。

将 k 值和 b 值代入 Hansch 方程，得到预测公式。根据预测公式，计算出预测值 $\log (1/IC_{50})$，将预测值和实验值的 $\log (1/IC_{50})$ 数据填入表 10 - 9，根据表中数据做散点图，经线性回归，得到回归方程和回归系数 R^2，最后根据上述的一系列结果对该系列化合物的构效关系进行讨论分析。

表 10 - 9　根据回归所得的 Hansch 方程及实测的 Log（$1/IC_{50}$）计算预测的 Log（$1/IC_{50}$）

3 - R_2 取代基	实测活性 Log（$1/IC_{50}$）	预测活性 Log（$1/IC_{50}$）
H		
F		
Cl		
Br		
I		
CH_3		
CH_2CH_3		
CH（CH_3）$_2$		
CH_2CH（CH_3）$_2$		
OCH_3		
OCH（CH_3）$_2$		
N（CH_3）$_2$		

三、实验报告要求

（一）化学合成部分

除了按正常要求和格式提供实验报告外，最后得到的化合物按 *Journal of Medicinal Chemistry* 的格式对实验结果进行描述，包括收率、数字化的红外及 NMR 数据。

（二）生物测试部分

包括初测和 IC_{50} 测试的加样表格、结果和数据处理所得到的图和表等。

（三）构效关系分析部分

通过 IC_{50} 值的实验数据对甲胺基和乙胺基 2 个系列化合物的构效关系进行定性分析；使用 Excel 软件对 IC_{50} 值的实验数据进行多元线性回归，分别拟合甲胺基和乙胺基 2 个系列化合物（只对 3 - 取代芳基系列化合物）的 Hansch 方程，评价拟合结果和进行定量构效关系分析，并根据该方程推测如何才能找到活性更好的化合物，给出该系列化合物的结构改造方向；对比实测数据和预测数据，通过图表的趋势分析结果的可靠性。

（四）数据处理

提交生物测试部分和构效关系分析部分的数据处理和图表结果的 Excel 文档（文件名：班级 + 姓名 + 学号）。

（五）总结

对实验总体进行讨论，写出总结报告。

四、附注

（1）推荐的展开系统为乙酸乙酯：石油醚 = 1 : 5，但不同的反应体系，需要根据初始的 TLC 结果对展开剂极性进行适当的调整。其中，甲氧基苯酚、3 - 二甲胺基苯酚推荐用乙酸乙酯：石油醚 = 1 : 3 洗脱。

（2）化合物在进行分析测试前，最好在真空下把残余的少量溶剂去除，以免溶剂对测试结果产生干扰。

（3）购买回来的乙酰胆碱酯酶为干粉状，活力单位数仅作为参考，并非确定值，用前先用缓冲液配成浓溶液（2.5 U/μL）并分装成若干管备用，可避免反复冻融。取一管稀释成系列酶浓度以测试活力，一般选取在该测试环境和测试条件下，最终的吸光度最大值不超过 2 为合适。酶的浓溶液在 5 ℃下可稳定保存 1 个星期以上。

（4）萘基、4 - 溴和 3 - 异丙基取代的化合物溶解度较低，可配成 2 mmol/L 的原液再稀释。

（5）使用排枪加入 DTNB + ATC 可避免逐个加样引起的时间差，使所有的样品都在同一时间启动反应。

（6）请参阅 Excel 中关于函数 LINEST 的具体说明和例子。

五、思考题

（1）以二甲氨基苯酚为原料进行反应时，为何后处理不可使用 HCl 溶液进行洗涤？

（2）在进行乙酰胆碱酯酶抑制活性测试时，所用酶的单位数、测试时间对结果有什么影响？还有哪些因素会对最终测试结果产生比较大的影响？

（3）如何解释实验测出的数据与文献报道数据之间的差异？

（4）为什么二甲氨基取代的产物在硅胶柱层析的时候拖尾比较严重？如何解决？

（5）对该系列化合物的构效关系进行全面分析，从取代基的取代位置、疏水性、电性和立体位阻等方面进行总结分析，通过 Hansch 方程结合具体例子进行说明。

Experiment 10　Synthesis of Aryl Alkylcarbamate, Activity Assay and Structure-Activity Relationships Analysis of Acetylcholinesterase Inhibitory

1. Learning Objectives

(1) To master two different esterification methods.

(2) To master the separation and purification technologies of silica gel column chromatography.

(3) To understand the principles and methods of AChE activity screening technology.

(4) To understand the methods and principles of structure-activity relationship analyses

2. Experimental Principles and Procedure

2.1　Synthesis of Aryl Alkylcarbamate

2.1.1　Experimental Principles

Method one: as shown in Figure 10 – 1.

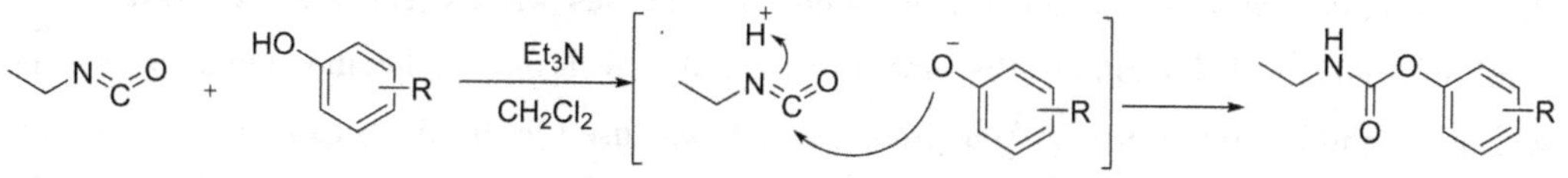

Figure 10 – 1　Synthesis of Alkylcarbamate (method one)

Method two: as shown in Figure 10 – 2.

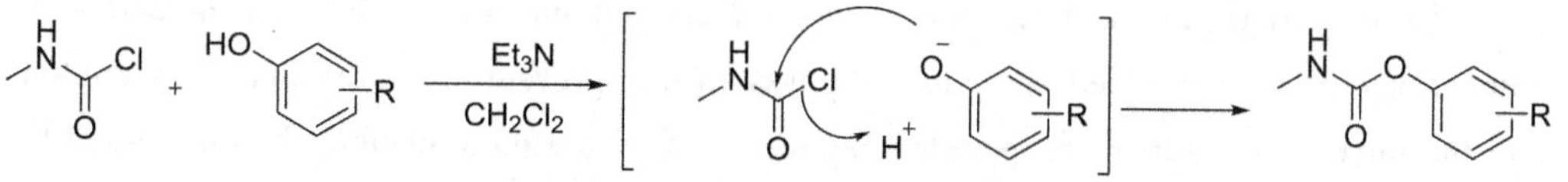

Figure 10 – 2　Synthesis of Alkylcarbamate (method two)

2.2　Experimental method

2.2.1　Experimental Reagents

The experimental reagents are shown in Table 10 – 1.

Table 10 – 1　Dosage and specifications of experimental reagents

Reagents	Grade	Intended Amount	Amount of Substance/mmol	Molar Ratio	Safety Data
Ethyl isocyanate (method one)	Analytical pure		9	1.5	
Methylcarbamoyl chloride (method two)	Analytical pure				

Table 10 − 1 (Continued)

Reagents	Grade	Intended Amount	Amount of Substance/mmol	Molar Ratio	Safety Data
Phenol	Analytical pure		6	1	
Triethylamine	Analytical pure		12	2	
Dichloromethane	Analytical pure	5 mL (method one) 10 mL (method two)			

Notes: other reagents include ethyl acetate, anhydrous caCl$_2$, anhydrous Na$_2$SO$_4$ sulphate, saturated brine, 4 mol/L HCl solution.

2. 2. 2　Methods

Method one: phenol (6 mmol) was added to a 50 mL reaction flask, dichloromethane (5 mL) and triethylamine (12 mmol) were added and mixed, and then ethyl isocyanate (9 mmol) was added. A drying tube was used to prevent moisture from accumulating, and the mixture was stirring at room temperature. TLC was used to monitor the progress of the reaction until the raw phenol disappeared (usually within 0. 5 − 1 h). After the reaction, 30 mL of dichloromethane was added, and the reaction solution was washed successively with water, 4 mL of 4 mol/L HCl solution (the product substituted with dimethylamino cannot be washed with acid) and saturated brine. Anhydrous Na$_2$SO$_4$ was used to dry the organic layer, and then the organic solvent was removed under reduced pressure. The residue can be placed in the same airtight container and stored until the next step.

Method two: phenol (6 mmol) was added to a 50 mL reaction flask, dichloromethane (10 mL) and triethylamine (12 mmol) were added and mixed, and then methylcarbamoyl chloride (9 mmol) was added. A drying tube was used to prevent moisture from accumulating, and the mixture was stirring at room temperature. TLC was used to monitor the progress of the reaction until the raw phenol disappeared (usually within 1 − 2 h). After the reaction, 30 mL of dichloromethane was added, and the reaction solution was washed successively with water, 4 mL of 4 mol/L HCl (the product substituted with dimethylamino cannot be washed with acid) and saturated brine. Anhydrous Na$_2$SO$_4$ was used to dry the organic layer, and then the organic solvent was removed under reduced pressure. The residue can be placed in the same airtight container and stored until the next step.

2. 2　Purification of Compounds

The crude product obtained in the previous step was dissolved in a small amount of dichloromethane and placed in a glass petri dish. Approximately 5 g of silica gel was added, and the sample was volatized in a fume hood with stirring until the silica gel was free of lumps and exhibited good fluidity. The ratio of the eluent was determined by thin layer chromatography (which generally required R_f of the substance to be separated is approximately 0.3). Another empty column was used for column chromatography, and approximately 20 – 30 g of silica gel (200 – 300 mesh) was placed into the column with the wet method. After equilibration, the sample was added for elution. TLC was used to check the separation of the sample. The components of the separated and purified product were combined. The purified product was obtained after being concentrated. The samples were sealed and stored for further use in the next analytical test.

Structural confirmation of compounds: the melting point, IR and ^{1}H-NMR data of the purified product were collected, and the structure was analyzed.

2.3　Activity Assay of the Compounds as Acetylcholinesterase Inhibitors

2.3.1　Experimental Principles

Activity assays of acetylcholinesterase (ACHE) inhibitors are based on Ellman's assay and involve ultraviolet spectroscopy. This assay works in the following way: AChE hydrolyzes the substrate acetylthiocholine (ATCI) and produces thiocholine. The thiocholine reacts with 5,5′-dithiobis-(2-nitrobenzoic acid) (DTNB) and produces 5-thio-2-nitrobenzoic acid with UV absorption at 412 nm. The rate of 5-thio-2-nitrobenzoic acid generation is positively correlated with the enzyme activity. The reaction process is shown in Figure 10 – 3.

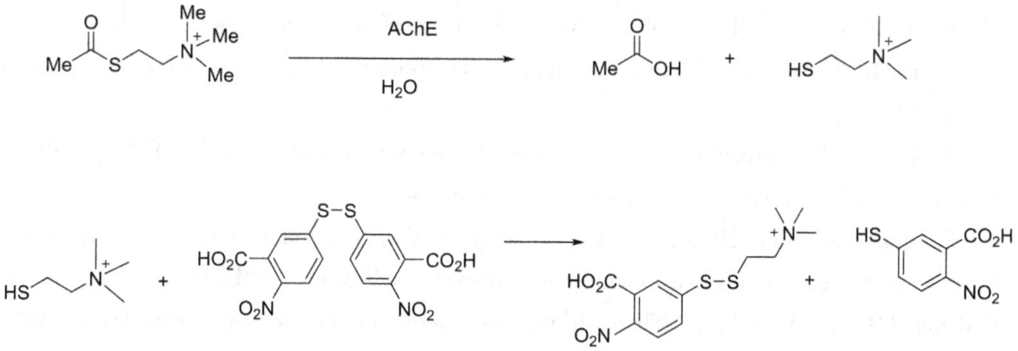

Figure 10 – 3　Experimental mechanism for the activity assay of acetylcholinesterase inhibitors

During the activity assay, the small molecule and AChE are within the system. After the substrate is added, the small molecule competes with the substrate for the enzymatic catalytic site. When the small molecule exerts inhibitory activity on the enzyme, substrate hydrolysis by the enzyme is reduced, and yellow 5-thio-2-nitrobenzoic acid is also reduced. Therefore, the UV absorption value at 412 nm is lower than that of the negative control. The lower the UV absorption value is, the better the inhibitory activity of the small molecule will be.

The half-maximal inhibitory concentration (IC_{50}) measures the effectiveness of a small molecule in inhibiting enzymes; the value refers to the concentration of an inhibitor in which the enzymatic activity, compared with its activity without an inhibitor, is reduced by half. Therefore, the smaller the IC_{50} is, the higher the inhibitory activity against the enzyme. Enzyme activity can be expressed by the rate of reaction catalyzed by an enzyme under certain conditions. The higher the reaction rate is, the greater the enzymatic activity will be, and the smaller the reaction rate is, the lower the enzymatic activity will be. In the experiment, the enzymatic activity can be measured by the rate of catalysis in the reaction. The reaction rate can be indicated by how much the substrate is reduced or how much the product is produced in a unit of time.

2.3.2 Method for Testing the Inhibitory Activity of AChE

(1) The buffer saline is prepared as follows:

A. Phosphate buffer saline (PBS; 0.1 mol/L, pH 8.0): mix 94 mL of 1.0 mol/L K_2HPO_4 solution with 6 mL of 1.0 mol/L KH_2PO_4 solution. Adjust the solution pH to 8.0 and dilute with deionized water to 1 000 mL. Store the samples at 4 ℃ for later use.

B. AChE solution (needs to be prepared before actual use): dilute a concentrated solution of AChE (approximately 2.5 U/μL) with 0.1 mol/L pH 8.0 PBS to 0.5 - 2 U/mL. The dilution ratio is based on the pre-determined activity.

C. Thioacetylcholine (ATC) solution (0.01 mol/L): weigh 31.6 mg of thioacetylcholine and dissolve it in 15.0 mL of 0.1 mol/L pH 8.0 PBS, then store the solution at 4 ℃ in the dark.

D. DTNB solution (0.01 mol/L): weigh 59.4 mg of DTNB and dissolve it in 15.0 mL of 0.1 mol/L pH 8.0 PBS. Aliquot the samples into brown EP tubes and store them in the dark at 4 ℃.

E. ATC + DTNB mixed solution: mix the previously prepared ATC and DTNB solutions at a ratio of 1:1 (prepare immediately before actual use).

F. Sample solution (50.0 mmol/L): weigh a certain amount of a sample for analysis and dissolve it in an appropriate amount of dimethyl sulfoxide (DMSO) to generate a 50.0 mmol/L sample solution. Then, dilute the sample to the desired concentration with 0.1 mol/L pH 8.0 PBS.

(2) Method.

A. Preliminary screening analysis: before performing the assay, dilute the 50 mmol/L sample solution with PBS to the create five gradient concentrations (2 mmol/L, 200 μmol/L, 20 μmol/L, 2 μmol/L and 0.2 μmol/L) (Figure 10 - 4). In a transparent 96-well plate, set up enzyme blank wells, DTNB blank wells and inhibitor wells of various concentrations respectively (setting up duplicate wells can reduce errors). Add the reagents according to the dosages shown in Table 10 - 2[except DTNB + ATC (1:1] mixture). The 96-well plate was covered and incubated at 37 ℃ for 10 min. After incubation, add the DTNB + ATC (1:1) mixture, and immediately use a microplate reader for detection. The microplate reader is set up as follows: automatic oscillation for 10 s. Read the UV absorption curve of each sample well at 412 nm, that is, the catalytic curve of the enzyme, and collect data within 3 min, with an interval of 15 s for each data point.

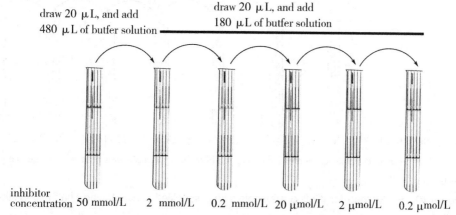

Figure 10 – 4　Dilution method for a sample with a specified concentration (1 : 10 dilution)

Table 10 – 2　Types and volumes of samples added to each well in the preliminary screening analysis

Reagents	Inhibitor					Enzyme blank	DTNB blank	Control
	2000 μmol/L	200 μmol/L	20 μmol/L	2 μmol/L	0.2 μmol/L			
Buffer/μL	20	20	20	20	20	100	90	80
Inhibitor/μL	60	60	60	60	60	0	0	0
DTNB/μL	0	0	0	0	0	0	10	0
AChE/μL	20	20	20	20	20	20	20	20
DTNB + ATC/μL	20	20	20	20	20	0	0	20
Total volume/μL	120	120	120	120	120	120	120	120
Final concentration /(μmol · L^{-1})	1 000	100	10	1	0.1			

Notes: the DTNB + ATC sample is added with a multichannel pipette. Buffer, inhibitor, DTNB, and AChE are added before incubation, while DNTB + ATC is added before measurement.

B. Determination of IC$_{50}$: determine the approximate range of inhibitory activity by utilizing the previous preliminary screening results. Set a series of compound concentrations (Figure 10 – 5) by half-fold dilution to cover the range of inhibitory activity of compounds. Prepare the test solution according to the reagents and doses shown in Table 10 – 3 (the test range and the number of test points can be increased or decreased as needed), and then follow the preliminary screening process to carry out the test.

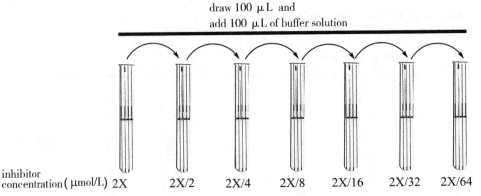

draw 100 μL and
add 100 μL of buffer solution

inhibitor
concentration(μmol/L) 2X   2X/2   2X/4   2X/8   2X/16   2X/32   2X/64

X represents the final concentration of the inhibitor in the sample well after adding the sample to the first well.

Figure 10 – 5   Method for diluting a sample with a specified concentration (half-fold dilution)

Table 10 – 3   Types and volumes of samples added to each well in IC_{50} analysis

Reagents	Inhibitor							Enzyme blank	DTNB blank	Control
	2 X μmol/L	2 X/2 μmol/L	2 X/4 μmol/L	2 X/8 μmol/L	2 X/16 μmol/L	2 X/32 μmol/L	2 X/64 μmol/L			
Buffer/μL	20	20	20	20	20	20	20	100	90	80
Inhibitor/μL	60	60	60	60	60	60	60	0	0	0
DTNB/μL	0	0	0	0	0	0	0	0	10	0
AChE/μL	20	20	20	20	20	20	20	20	20	20
DTNB + ATC	20	20	20	20	20	20	20	0	0	20
Total volume/μL	120	120	120	120	120	120	120	120	120	120
Final concentration / (μmol/L^{-1})	X	X/2	X/4	X/8	X/16	X/32	X/64			

Notes: the DTNB + ATC sample is added with a multichannel pipette. Buffer, inhibitor, DTNB, and AChE are added before incubation, while DNTB + ATC is added before measurement.

C. Data processing: the DTNB blank is used as the experimental background. Subtract the value of the DTNB blank from the data of the enzyme control and the small molecule inhibitor to obtain a value. Draw the resulting value against time. The points of each series are linearly fitted to obtain the equation $y = Kx + B$. The slope, K, represents the relative activity of the enzyme (Table 10 – 4), and the inhibitory activity of the small molecule inhibitor can be calculated with the following formula:

$$\text{Inhibition rate } (\%) = (1 - K_{\text{inhibitor}}/K_{\text{enzyme}}) \times 100\%$$

Table 10 −4　Calculating the IC_{50} value for the AChE inhibitory activity of the compounds

Concentration	X μmol/L	X/2 μmol/L	X/4 μmol/L	X/8 μmol/L	X/16 μmol/L
K_{enzyme}					
$K_{inhibitor}$					
Inhibition rate/%					
$IC_{50}/(\mu mol\cdot L^{-1})$					

Origin, SPSS or GraphPad Prism software can be used for data processing. Make a scatter plot chart for Log $C_{inhibitor}$ and the inhibition rate (%), and use nonlinear regression to obtain the IC_{50}. Finally, record the test data from your experiments and other classmates in Table 10 −5 (Data for the same compound in different tests should be averaged).

Table 10 −5　Summary of the IC_{50} result for the AChE inhibitory activity of several compounds

R₂	$R_1 = -CH_3$		$R_1 = -C_2H_5$	
	Measured IC_{50} /(μmol· L⁻¹)	Theoretical IC_{50} /(μmol· L⁻¹)	Measured IC_{50} /(μmol· L⁻¹)	Theoretical IC_{50} /(μmol· L⁻¹)
− H	200			
2 − Br	2. 2			
2 − i − Pr	6. 0			
3 − F	85			
3 − Cl	50			
3 − Br	13			
3 − I	7. 0			
3 − CH_3	14			
3 − C_2H_5	4. 8			
3 − i − Pr	0. 34			
3 − OCH_3	22			
3 − i − OPr	9. 2			
3 − N (CH_3)₂	8			

Table 10 – 5 (Continued)

R₂	$R_1 = -CH_3$		$R_1 = -C_2H_5$	
	Measured IC_{50} /(μmol· L^{-1})	Theoretical IC_{50} /(μmol· L^{-1})	Measured IC_{50} /(μmol· L^{-1})	Theoretical IC_{50} /(μmol· L^{-1})
4 – Br		88		
4 – CH₃		—		
4 – i – Pr		70		
4 – OCH₃		80		
Ar = – 1 – naphthyl		0. 9		
Ar = -2-naphthyl		14		
3, 5-diMe		6. 0		

2. 4   Analysis of the Structure-Activity Relationships

2. 4. 1   Experiment Principles

The quantitative structure-activity relationship (QSAR) provides information on the relationship between the biological activity and structural characteristics of a group of compounds. Structural characteristics are represented by physical and chemical parameters, molecular topological parameters, quantum chemical indices and structural fragmentation indices. In QSAR, a mathematical statistics method is used to perform data regression analysis, and the pattern of quantitative changes with mathematical models are obtained. The QSAR is defined as 2D-QSAR since its mathematical models are derived from the two-dimensional structures of compounds.

Hansch-Fujita correlation analysis is the most commonly used structure-activity relationship analysis method in 2D-QSAR. This method is based on the principal that drugs transport *in vivo* and that the interactions of drugs and receptors are governed by physical and chemical interactions between drug molecules and biological macromolecules. Drugs must pass through several biofilms and a certain number of lipid-water interfaces from the drug delivery site to the target. Therefore, drug transport is related to the partition coefficient, and the potency of a drug is affected by its concentration when it reaches the target. Biological activity is exerted by the interactions of drugs with targets through covalent bonds, ionic bonds, ion-dipole bonds, hydrogen bonds, hydrophobic bonds, chelation, and van der Waals forces, etc. These interactions are related to the chemical structure, electronic effect, and steric effect of drug molecules. Thus, as proposed by Hansch, the biological activity of homologs and the physicochemical parameters of various substituents are correlated. This correlation is expressed by the following parametric equation (Hansch equation) , which is related to free energy.

$$Log\ (1/C)\ =\ -\ k_1\pi^2\ +\ k_2\pi\ +\ k_3\sigma\ +\ k_4\ MR\ +\ k_5$$

where C is the molar concentration of a certain compound that produces a certain effect; π is a measure of the hydrophobicity; σ is a measure of the hydrophobicity electronic effects; MR is a measure of steric factors; k_1, k_2, k_3 and k_4 represent the weight coefficients of the contributions of various factors, which are related to the compounds and assay conditions (Table 10 - 6). These measures are obtained by the least square method and multiple regression analysis.

Table 10 -6   Representative parameters of substituents on the aromatic ring

- R	π	σ_m	MR
H	0. 00	0. 00	1. 03
F	0. 14	0. 34	0. 92
Cl	0. 71	0. 37	6. 03
Br	0. 86	0. 39	8. 88
I	1. 12	0. 35	13. 94
CH_3	0. 56	- 0. 07	5. 65
CH_2CH_3	1. 02	- 0. 07	10. 30
$CH(CH_3)_2$	1. 53	- 0. 07	14. 98
$CH_2CH(CH_3)_2$	1. 98	- 0. 10	19. 62
OCH_3	- 0. 02	0. 12	7. 87
$OCH(CH_3)_2$	0. 36	0. 10	17. 06
$N(CH_3)_2$	0. 18	- 0. 15	15. 55

(1) Hydrophobicity parameters. The hydrophobic parameter π is characterized by the logarithm Log P of the lipid-water partition coefficient P of the drug molecule as follows:

$$\pi_x\ =\ Log\ P_x\ -\ Log\ P_H$$

where Log P_H is the lipid-water partition coefficient of the unsubstituted compound, Log P_x is the lipid-water partition coefficient of the compound substituted by X. When π is positive, it means that the group exhibits a greater lipophilicity than that of a hydrogen substituent, and the negative π means the group exhibits a greater hydrophilicity than that of a hydrogen substituent. The π values can be found in Table 10 - 6, which were determined by equation calculation with chromatographic parameter R, or calculated through software.

(2) Electrical parameters. The influence of the electronic effects of substituents on the molecular reactivity can be measured by the Hammett constant (σ) in the Hammett equation. The σ value of a substituent reflects the sum of inductive and conjugative effects. In the para position, these two kinds of effects occur simultaneously. In the meta position, there are only inductive effects. In the ortho position, in addition to the above two kinds of effects, there are also ortho position effects caused by steric hindrance or hydrogen bonds; hence, σ needs to be handled specifically. A positive σ indicates an electron-withdrawing group, and a negative σ indicates an electron-donating group. The σ values can be found in Table 10 – 6.

(3) Stereo parameters. Multiple parameters can be used to characterize the steric factors of substituents. Here, the factors are characterized by the molar refractivity, which is defined as follows:

$$MR = [(n^2 - 1)/(n^2 + 2)](MW/d)$$

where n is the liquid refractive index, MW is the molecular weight, d is the density, and MW/d is the molar volume of the liquid. The MR value of an atom or a group can be obtained from the MR of a molecule. The negative MR in the equation means that steric hindrance is the main influencing factor, while the positive MR means that the dispersion force generated by induced polarization is the main influencing factor. MR values can be found in Table 10 – 6.

Hansch analysis is only used for homologs with the same mechanism of action, i. e. a series of compounds that contain the same basic structure but different substituents. When designing compounds, the substituents should be selected so that their physical and chemical parameters exhibit a certain range of change from negative to positive and the biological activity data also show a large difference (at least one logarithmic unit or more). The number of compounds is generally at least five times the number of physical and chemical parameters to ensure the accuracy of statistical results.

Hansch analysis is processed by multiple linear regression (MLR), and the coefficient of each dependent variable is obtained by the least square method to generate the regression equation. To study QSARs using this method, the correlation between the parameters must be small or nonexistent, that is, each parameter represents an independent variable in the equation.

2.4.2 QSAR Analysis

According to the Hansch equation:

$$\text{Log}(1/C) = -k_1\pi^2 + k_2\pi + k_3\sigma + k_4 MR + k_5$$

The parameters substituent group listed in Table 10 – 6 and corresponding IC_{50} values are listed in Table 10 – 7. Use the LINEST function ([known_y's], [known_x's], [const], [stats]) in Excel to perform linear regression, in which [known_y's] corresponds to log (1/IC_{50}); [known_x's] corresponds to π^2, π, σ_m and MR; [const] takes the TRUE value; and [stats] takes the TRUE value. Copy the formula to a blank worksheet and then select a 5×5

range of cells that begins with the formula cell. Press F2, then press *Ctrl + Shift + Enter*. If the formula is not entered as an array formula, a single result will be returned. When inputting data as an array, the regression statistics results will be returned, which can be used to identify the desired statistical value. The parameter meanings corresponding to the results of the regression statistics are shown in Table 10 – 8.

Table 10 – 7   Parameter data for Hansch analysis
(QSAR analysis is performed only for 3 – R_2 substituents)

3 – R_2	IC_{50}(μmol/L)	$1/IC_{50}$	log ($1/IC_{50}$)	π^2	π	σ_m	MR
H							
F							
Cl							
Br							
I							
CH_3							
CH_2CH_3							
$CH(CH_3)_2$							
$CH_2CH(CH_3)_2$							
OCH_3							
$OCH(CH_3)_2$							
$N(CH_3)_2$							

Table 10 – 8   The parameters corresponding to the output results of the LINEST function

k_4	k_3	k_2	k_1	b
se_4	se_3	se_2	se_1	se_b
r^2	Se_y			
F	D_f			
ss_{reg}	Ss_{resid}			

Notes: the *k* values correspond to the coefficients before each parameter of the Hansch equation (the order given in Excel is reversed). The *se* values are the standard deviation of the corresponding coefficients. Se_y is the standard error of the *y* estimates. r^2 is the coefficient of determination, i. e. the ratio of the estimated value of *y* to the actual value. The better a model is at making predictions, the closer the r^2 value will be to 1. *F* is the *F* statistic, which can be used to determine whether there is an occasional observable relationship between the dependent variable and the independent variable. D_f is the degrees of freedom, which can be used to find the *F* critical value on a statistical table. ss_{reg} is the regression sum of squares. Ss_{resid} is the residual sum of squares.

Substitute the k value and b value into the Hansch equation to obtain the prediction formula. Based on the prediction formula, calculate the predicted Log $(1/IC_{50})$, fill in the predicted and measured value of Log $(1/IC_{50})$ in Table $10-9$, and generate a scatter plot. Obtain the regression equation and coefficient R^2 by linear regression. Finally, analyze and discuss the structure-activity relationship of this series of compounds according to the above results.

Table 10 – 9   According to the obtained Hansch equation and the measured Log($1/IC_{50}$), calculate the predicted Log($1/IC_{50}$)

$3 - R_2$	Measured Log $(1/IC_{50})$	Predicted Log $(1/IC_{50})$
H		
F		
Cl		
Br		
I		
CH_3		
CH_2CH_3		
$CH(CH_3)_2$		
$CH_2CH(CH_3)_2$		
OCH_3		
$OCH(CH_3)_2$		
$N(CH_3)_2$		

3. Experimental report requirements

3.1   Chemical Synthesis

In addition to providing the experimental report, the final products should be described in the format of *Journal of Medicinal Chemistry*, including the product yield, digital infrared spectra and NMR data.

3.2   Biological Assay

Provide the sample adding tables, the experimental results and the graphs and tables obtained from processed the data from the preliminary screening analysis and IC_{50} analysis.

3.3   Structure-Activity relationship analysis

The structure-activity relationship of the compounds substituted by methylamine groups and ethylamine groups was qualitatively analyzed through the IC_{50} experimental data. Excel was used to perform multiple linear regression on the IC_{50} experimental data. The Hansch equation of the two kinds of compounds above was fit, and the fitting results were evaluated and the QSAR analyzed. Speculate on a way to discover compounds that exhibit better activity according to the equation and conceive the direction in which this series of compounds should be structurally modified. Compare the measured data are with the predicted data, and analyze the reliability of the results through the trend in the chart.

3.4　Data Processing

Submit the Excel document of the data processing and graph results for the biological assay part and the structure-activity relationship analysis part (file name: class + name + student number).

3.5　Discussion

Discuss the overall experiment and write a summary report.

4. Notes

(1) The recommended developing solvent system is ethyl acetate : petroleum ether = 1 : 5, while its polarity must be adjusted appropriately for different reaction systems according to the initial thin layer results. Among the compounds, methoxyphenol and 3-dimethylaminophenol are recommended to be eluted with ethyl acetate : petroleum ether = 1 : 3.

(2) The residual solvent should be removed under vacuum before analyzing and testing the compounds to prevent the solvent from interfering with the test results.

(3) The purchased AChE is dry powder, and the units of activity are only for reference, not a definite value. A concentrated solution (2.5 U/μL) was prepared with buffer solution and divided into several tubes before use to avoid repeated freezing and thawing. The stock solution was diluted into a series of different enzyme concentrations to test the activity. It is preferable that the final maximum absorbance does not exceed 2 under the test environment and conditions. The concentrated solution can be stored for at least one week at 5 ℃.

(4) The solubility of naphthyl-, 4-bromo- and 3-isopropyl-substituted compounds is low, so they were prepared into 2 mmol/L stock solutions before dilution.

(5) The DTNB + ATC mixed solution should be added by multichannel pipettes to avoid the time difference, which is caused by adding samples one by one, so that all samples start the reaction simultaneously.

(6) Please refer to the specific descriptions and examples of the LINEST function in Excel.

5. Questions

(1) When using dimethyl aminophenol as the raw material of the reaction, why cannot HCl be used to wash the solution in post-processing?

(2) In the AChE inhibitory activity assay, how do the units of enzyme and the test time

affect the results? What other factors have an impact on the final test results?

(3) How can we explain the discrepancy between the experimentally measured data and the data reported in the literature?

(4) Why does the dimethylamino-substituted product undergo serious tailing during silica gel column chromatography, and what is the solution?

(5) Comprehensively analyze the structure-activity relationship of this series of compounds in regard to the position of the substituents as well as the hydrophobicity, electricity and steric hindrance of the substituents through the Hansch equation, and include specific examples.

References

[1] LOCOCK K, TRAN H, CODD R, et al. Hands-On approach to structure activity relationships: the synthesis, testing, and hansch analysis of a series of acetylcholineesterase inhibitors [J]. Journal of chemical education, 2015, 92 (10): 1745 – 1750.

[2] ELLMAN G L, COURTNEY K D, ANDRES V, et al. A new and rapid colorimetric determination of acetylcholinesterase activity[J]. Biochemical pharmacology, 1961, 7: 88 – 95.

[3] 付伟, 叶德泳. 计算机辅助药物设计导论[M]. 2 版. 北京: 化学工业出版社, 2017.

实验十一　白藜芦醇的合成（设计性实验）

一、实验目的

（1）提高学生综合运用基础知识和基本技能的能力。

（2）培养学生学习设计性实验的基本思路，学会科学的试验组合，提出合理的实验方案。

（3）加强学生观察实验现象、准确记录实验数据、正确处理分析和总结实验结果的技能。

（4）培养学生查阅资料和撰写科学论文的能力。

（5）培养学生的科研素养、科研思维、科研技能、科研道德等。

（6）培养学生团结互助的团体精神和组织协调能力，培养学生的责任心、计划性和探索精神。

（7）培养学生的科研素养和创新能力，使学生具有从事本专业实际工作和研究工作的初步能力。

二、实验要求

（1）课程负责教师须提前4个月向学生介绍课程的性质、任务、要求、课程安排和进度、实验守则及实验室安全制度等。

（2）实验课程以开放探索实验为主，学生利用课余时间选定题目，查阅、分析相关文献，在实验开始前2个月时，制作相应的PPT并与带课教师一起讨论，制定合理可行的实验方案及合成路线，并自己准备实验内容和提交实验材料计划。

（3）带课教师根据讨论后确定的实验方案准备实验材料。

（4）实验时间在规定的时间段为开放性的，学生在实验前必须进行预习，由学生操作完成实验，操作和实验记录需规范，数据需真实可靠，对实验结果应进行认真总结和讨论。

（5）实验过程中，教师应在实验室进行巡视，及时纠正学生的错误操作，检查学生的预习报告和实验记录，引导学生独立分析和解决问题。

（6）实验报告要求学生以原始记录为基础，以书面形式翔实叙述每次实验的目的、原理、操作过程、现象和结果等，并以讨论的形式如实叙述实验过程中发现的问题、个人的体会及实验的注意事项等。每次实验报告应包含以下内容：实验题目、实验目的、实验原理、实验内容、实验结果及讨论。

（7）每个实验结束，教师要对学生在实验过程中出现的问题进行总结和讨论，鼓励学生对实验提出自己的建议，尤其要对失败的实验进行深刻总结，并找出失败的原因。实验结束时，课程的负责教师还要进行一次讨论和总结。

（8）阶段性实验完成后学生需要提交阶段性实验报告，内容包括实验的目的和意义、实验方案、实验原理及选取依据、参考文献、讨论记录、实验材料、实验实施情况及记录、实验结果及分析、实验体会讨论等。另外，整个实验完成后，学生必须提交一份实验总结。

三、实验方案的设计

（一）背景知识

白藜芦醇（resveratrol）（图 11 – 1）于 1963 年在何首乌根中被首次发现，但真正让其扬名世界的是 1989 年 WTO 所主持的一项流行病学调查，该调查证实法国人冠心病的发病率和死亡率比其他西方国家人群，尤其是比美国人和英国人要低得多。尽管法国人摄入的饱和脂肪酸几乎是美国人和英国人的 4 倍，但法国人罹患心脏病的危险却只是后者的1/3，这一现象被称为"法国悖论"。研究表明，此现象与法国是全球最大的葡萄酒生产和消费国密切相关。因为在优质的葡萄酒中存在白藜芦醇，其对人体具有重要的保健功能。目前，白藜芦醇可以作为药品、食品和保健品及美容护肤品来使用，其用途的多样性给实验研究带来广阔的空间。

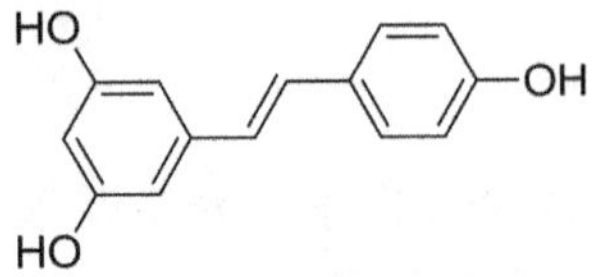

图 11 –1　白藜芦醇

（二）实验步骤

1. 作业

（1）数据库的使用，文献的查阅。
（2）设计合成路线。
（3）设计实验方案。
（4）制作 PPT 课件。
（5）上交综述和实验方案材料。

2. 实验前讨论

（1）PPT 演示和讨论。

（2）提出修改意见，确定实验方案。

（3）总结讨论结果。

（4）根据实验方案进行实验准备。

3. 实验和阶段性总结

（1）基本知识点和注意事项的讲解。

（2）对实验中可能出现问题的分析和处理。

（3）实验的进行，观察和记录。

（4）备用方案。

（5）结构的测定和解析。

4. 课程总结和讨论

（1）PPT 展示实验结果。

（2）产品的提交和验收。

（3）对实验过程中出现问题的讲解和分析。

（4）数据的分析和总结。

（5）仪器的检查验收。

（6）报告的验收。

（三）实验仪器、试剂和材料

1. 仪器设备

玻璃仪器，烘箱，磁力搅拌器，微波反应仪，电热套，电炉，三用紫外分析仪，紫外分光光度计，红外分光光度计，核磁共振波谱仪，液质联用仪，制冰机，旋转蒸发仪，真空水泵，红外干燥箱，电子天平，油泵，冰柜，无水溶剂制备装置，层析缸。

另外，根据同学们的具体设计方案进行仪器的准备，并在课前调试到可使用的状态，新仪器要进行必要的培训才可上机操作。

2. 可能用到的试剂与材料

二氯甲烷，乙醚，甲醇，乙酸乙酯，N,N-二甲基苯胺，吡啶，无水 1，2-二氯乙烷，N，N-二甲基甲酰胺，三乙胺，四氢呋喃，乙醇，无水 Na_2SO_4，无水 $MgSO_4$，无水 $CaCl_2$，$NaCl$，无水 Na_2CO_3，$NaHSO_3$，无水 $AlCl_3$，$NaOH$，KBr（测红外压片用），吡啶盐酸盐，甲醇钠，乙醇钠，叔丁醇钾，NaH，CaH_2，BBr_3，对甲氧基甲苯，3，5-二甲氧基甲苯，对甲氧基苄醇，3，5-二甲氧基苄醇，对羟基苯乙酸，3，5-二甲氧基苯乙酸，3，5-二羟基苯甲醛，对甲氧基苯甲醛，3，5-二甲氧基苯甲醛，四丁基碘化铵，羟甲基纤维素钠，薄层硅胶 G，薄层板，喹啉，铜粉，HBr，PBr_3，亚磷酸三乙酯，氘代溶剂。

真空脂，注射器，橡胶塞，氧气袋，分子筛，气球，核磁管。

具体的试剂种类和用量还要根据同学们设计的方案所涉及的试剂和材料提前进行

准备。

四、关键词

（1）白藜芦醇。
（2）逆反应合成策略。
（3）维蒂希反应。
（4）维蒂希－霄钠尔反应。
（5）珀金反应。
（6）格氏反应。
（7）赫克反应。
（8）酚类化合物的保护与脱保护策略。

五、建议

详细了解每类反应的机制和注意事项，比较应用不同类型的反应合成白藜芦醇时的优缺点。反应条件具体化时，注意多参考不同文献以做出合理的选择。开阔思维，勇于创新，将一些新反应、新技术应用于白藜芦醇的合成。

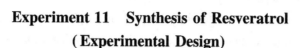

Experiment 11　Synthesis of Resveratrol
（Experimental Design）

1　Learning Objectives

（1）To improve the students' abilities to comprehensively employ their basic knowledge and skills.

（2）To train students to learn about the basic principles of experimental design, grouping scientifically and proposing rational experimental schemes.

（3）To improve students' several skills, including observing experimental phenomena, recording data precisely, analyzing correctly and summarizing the results.

（4）To train students' abilities to consult information and write scientific papers.

（5）To train students' scientific attainments, scientific intelligence, scientific skills and scientific integrity.

（6）To train students to promote group cooperation and a spirit of exploration, as well as the ability to organize, take on responsibilities and plan.

（7）To train students' scientific literacy and innovation abilities and the basic abilities perform practical works and research works.

2　Basic Requirements

（1）The teacher overseeing this course must introduce the substance, tasks, requirements, course arrangements and progress, rules and laboratory safety regulation to the students four months ahead.

（2）This experiment course is mainly for exploration experiments. Students must design their experiments in their spare time, consult and analyze relevant literature, and make a PPT to discuss with the teacher two months before the experiment. In this discussion, a feasible experimental scheme and synthesis route will be determined and the experimental preparation and experimental material plan will be submitted.

（3）The teacher will prepare the experimental materials according to the scheme obtained after the discussion.

（4）The experimental time is set in a specific period. Students must prepare before the experiments and finish the experiments by themselves. Operations and experimental records should meet the standards, and the data should be reliable. The results must be summarized and discussed.

（5）During the experimental process, the teacher should inspect the laboratory to correct the students' errors, examine their preparation reports and records, and guide them to analyze and solve problems independently.

(6) Students' reports must be based on their original records and the purposes, principles, operations, phenomena and results must be recorded with detail and accuracy in written form. In addition, the problems that occurred, personal experience and problems that should be noticed must be recorded in a discussion. The reports for each time should include experiment titles, purposes, principles, contents, the results and discussions.

(7) When an experiment is finished, the teacher should summarize and discuss the problems that occurred during students' experiments and encourage them to propose their suggestions for the experiments. Failed experiments must especially be summarized to determine the reasons for failure. After all experiments are finished, the teacher should conduct one more discussion and summarization.

(8) Experiment reports for each stage should be submitted once the experiment of each stage is finished, which includes the experiment purposes and significance, schemes, principles and their bases, reference, discussions, materials, progress and records, the results and analysis, experience discussion, etc. In addition, students should submit an experiment summarization after all sections are finished.

3　Design of the Experimental Protocol

3.1　Introduction

Resveratrol (Figure 11 – 1) was first found in the roots of *Polygonum multiflorum* in 1963. However, resveratrol became known worldwide through an epidemiological investigation hosted by the WTO in 1989, which demonstrated that the morbidity and mortality due to coronary heart disease were lower among individuals in France than other Western countries, especially America and Britain. Although saturated fatty acids were consumed almost four times more often by French compared to American and British, morbidity due to heart diseases in French was merely one-third than that of Americans and British. This phenomenon was called "the French Paradox". The research claimed that this phenomenon was closely related to the fact that the French are the largest wine producer and seller in the world. Fine wine contains resveratrol, which plays an important health role in the human body. Currently, resveratrol can be used in drugs, food, health care products, and skincare products. Its application diversity brings up broad possibilities for research.

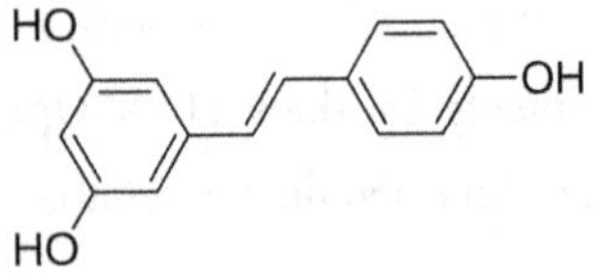

Figure 11 –1　Resveratrol

3.2　Experimental Procedures

3.2.1　Homework

(1) Use databank and consult literature.

(2) Design synthesis routes.

(3) Design an experiment scheme.

(4) Make a PPT.

(5) Submit the review and experimental scheme materials.

3.2.2　Discussion Before Experiments

(1) Present the PPT and discuss the experiment.

(2) Propose advice for revision and confirm the experimental scheme.

(3) Summarize the discussion results.

(4) Make preparations according to the experimental scheme.

3.2.3　Experiments and Summarization in Stages

(1) Explain the basic knowledge points and precautions.

(2) Analyze and solve problems may meet in experiments.

(3) Experiments, observe and record.

(4) Backup scheme.

(5) Test and analysis of structures.

3.2.4　Course Summary and Discussion

(1) Show experimental results by PPT.

(2) Submit and examine the products.

(3) Explain and analyze the problems in experiments.

(4) Analyze the data and conclude the results.

(5) Check the apparatus.

(6) Submit the reports.

4　Experimental Apparatus, Reagents and Materials

4.1　Experiment Apparatus

Glassware, drying oven, magnetic stirrer, microwave reactor, electric heater, electric stove, ultraviolet analyzer, ultraviolet spectrophotometer, infrared spectrophotometer, nuclear magnetic resonance spectrometer, liquid chromatograph mass spectrometer (LC-MS), ice maker, rotary evaporator, vacuum water pump, infrared dryer, electronic scales, oil pump, fridge, preparation device for water-free solvent, chromatographic tank.

In addition, apparatus is prepared based on students' scheme designs and becomes usable before class. Necessary training is needed before operating the new apparatus.

4.2　Possible Reagents and Materials

Dichloromethane, diethyl ether, methanol, ethyl acetate, N, N-dimethylaniline, pyridine, anhydrous 1, 2-dichloroethane, *N*, *N*-dimethylformamide, triethylamine, tetrahydrofuran, ethanol, anhydrous NaSO$_4$, anhydrous MgSO$_4$, anhydrous CaCl$_2$, NaCl, anhydrous Na$_2$CO$_3$, NaHSO$_3$, anhydrous AlCl$_3$, NaOH, KBr (for infrared tablets), pyridine hydrochloride, sodium methoxide, sodium ethoxide, potassium tert-butoxide, NaH, CaH$_2$, BBr$_3$, p-methoxytoluene, 3, 5-dimethoxytoluene, p-methoxybenzyl alcohol, 3, 5-dimethoxybenzyl alcohol, p-hydroxyphenylacetic acid, 3, 5-dimethoxyphenylacetic acid, 3, 5-dihydroxybenzaldehyde, p-methoxybenzaldehyde, 3, 5-dimethoxybenzaldehyde, tetrabutylammonium iodide, sodium carboxymethyl cellulose, thin layer silica gel G, thin layer plate, quinoline, copper powder, hydrobromic acid, PBr$_3$, triethyl phosphite, deuterated solvents.

Vacuum grease, syringe, rubber stopper, oxygen bag, molecular sieve, balloon, NMR tube.

Specific reagent types and scales were prepared according to students' scheme designs.

5   Key Words

(1) Resveratrol.

(2) Reverse reaction synthesis strategy.

(3) Wittig reaction.

(4) Wittig-Horner reaction.

(5) Perkin reaction.

(6) Grinard reaction.

(7) Heck reaction.

(8) Protection and deprotection of phenol compounds.

6   Helpful Tips

Learn about the mechanism and precautions of each type of reaction and compare the advantages and disadvantages of different types of reactions to synthesize resveratrol. When specifying the reaction conditions, refer to different studies to make one reasonable choice. Be open-minded and innovative, try to apply new reactions and new technologies to the synthesis of resveratrol.

附　录
Appendix

附录 **1**　实验报告的书写范例

时间（Date）：YYMMDD　　温度（Temp）：　　℃　　湿度（Humidity）：

1. 题目（Title）

2. 实验目的（Learning Objectives）

3. 反应式（Reaction Equations）

4. 原料与产物理化性质（Physical and Chemical Properties of Raw Materials and Products）

实验预习（Prelab）

名称 （Name）	分子式 （Molecular Formular）	分子量 （Molecular Weight）	晶型与颜色 （Crystal Type and Color）	沸点或熔点 （b. p. or m. p.）	密度 （Density）	溶解度 （Solubility）

5. 拟操作流程（Proposed Operation Process）

6. 原料、规格、用量与配比（Materials, Grade, Intended Amount and Ratio）

原料 （Materials）	规格 （Grade）	用量（重量或 体积）（Intended amount）	物质的量/Molar Amount of Substance/mmol	摩尔比 （Molar Ratio）	安全信息 （Safety Data）

实验中（In the Experiment）

7. 实验操作与现象（Procedure Including Observations and Work-Up）

时间（Time）	实验操作 （Experimental Procedure）	实验现象 （Phenomenon）
HH：MM		

（续上表）

8. 结果（Results）

产物 （Product）	外观 （Appearance）	得量 （Mass）	理论得量 （Theoretic Quantity）	收率 （Yield）	熔点 （m. p.）

粘贴 UV、IR 及 NMR 图谱，并对图谱进行结构解析。（Paste the UV, IR and NMR spectra, and analyze the structure according to the spectra.）

9. 讨论（Discussions）

（1）对实验某些现象进行解释，如果有文献依据，请标出文献出处。（Explain some phenomena in the experiment, if there are literature evidences, please cite the literatures.）

（2）本实验哪些操作不到位？（What operational errors were there in this experiment?）

（3）结合实验得到的图谱、薄层结果和熔点等信息，对实验的操作过程、产物的收率和纯度、可能的影响因素和可改进的内容进行综合分析。（Combined with the experimental spectra, TLC results, melting point, and other information, comprehensively analyze the experimental operation process, the yield and purity of the product, the possible influencing factors and improving contents.）

10. 思考题的回答（Answer the Questions）

课后（Postlab）

附录 2　危险品货物包装标签（GB 190—2009）

			爆炸性物质或物品	
爆炸性物质或物品			毒性物质	感染性物质
毒性气体	易燃气体		非易燃无毒气体	
易燃液体		易燃固体	易于自燃的物质	腐蚀性物质
遇水放出易燃气体的物质		有机过氧化物		氧化性物质
一级放射性物质	二级放射性物质	三级放射性物质	裂变性物质	杂项危险物质和物品

附录3　全球化学品统一分类和标签制度

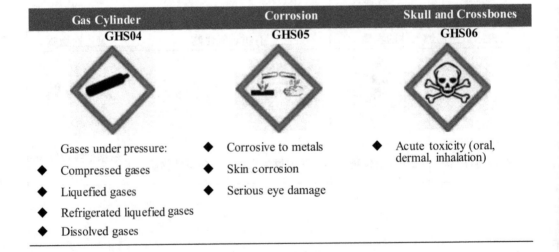

Exploding Bomb GHS01	Flame GHS02	Flame Over Circle GHS03

- Unstable explosives
- Explosives
- Self-reactive substances and mixtures
- Organic peroxides
- Fire or projection hazard
- May mass explode in fire

- Flammable gases
- Flammable aerosols
- Flammable liquids
- Flammable solids
- Self-reactive substances and mixtures
- Pyrophoric liquids
- Pyrophoric solids
- Self-heating substances and mixtures
- Substances and mixtures, which in contact with water
- Emit flammable gases
- Organic peroxides

- Oxidizing gases
- Oxidizing liquids

Gas Cylinder GHS04	Corrosion GHS05	Skull and Crossbones GHS06

Gases under pressure:
- Compressed gases
- Liquefied gases
- Refrigerated liquefied gases
- Dissolved gases

- Corrosive to metals
- Skin corrosion
- Serious eye damage

- Acute toxicity (oral, dermal, inhalation)

Exclamation Mark	Health Hazard	Environment
GHS07	GHS08	GHS09

- Acute toxicity (oral, dermal, inhalation)
- Skin irritation
- Eye irritation
- Skin sensitisation
- Specific target organ toxicity

- Respiratory sensitization
- Germ cell mutagenicity
- Carcinogenicity
- Reproductive toxicity
- Specific target organ toxicity-single exposure
- Specific target organ toxicity-repeated exposure
- Aspiration hazard

Hazardous to the aquatic environment:
- Acute hazard
- Chronic hazard

常用试剂化学品安全技术说明书（Material Safety Data Sheet，MSDS）查询网址：

◆ Chemical book：https：//msds.chemicalbook.com/

◆ Sigma 公司化学品安全技术说明书（MSDS）查询网址：https：//www.sigmaaldrich.com/china-mainland.html

◆ International labour organization：https：//www.ilo.org/dyn/icsc/showcard.listCards3？p_lang = zh

◆ 中国化学安全网：http：//service.nrcc.com.cn/tool/msds？SearchItem = 0

◆ 化源网：https：//www.chemsrc.com/MSDSIndex/

◆ Centers for Disease Control and Prevention：https：//www.cdc.gov/niosh/npg/

◆ MSDS 查询网址：http：//msds.anquan.com.cn/

附录4 常见有机溶剂作为痕量杂质
的 ^{1}H-NMR 和 ^{13}C-NMR 化学位移

^{1}H-NMR Data

Solvent	proton	mult	CDCl$_3$	(CD$_3$)$_2$CO	(CD$_3$)$_2$SO	C$_6$D$_6$	CD$_3$CN	CD$_3$OD	D$_2$O
Solvent residual peak			7.26	2.05	2.50	7.16	1.94	3.31	4.79
H$_2$O		s	1.56	2.84	3.33	0.40	2.13	4.87	
Acetic acid	CH$_3$	s	2.10	1.96	1.91	1.55	1.96	1.99	2.08
Acetone	CH$_3$	s	2.17	2.09	2.09	1.55	2.08	2.15	2.22
Acetonitrile	CH$_3$	s	2.10	2.05	2.07	1.55	1.96	2.03	2.06
Benzene	CH	s	7.36	7.36	7.37	7.15	7.37	7.33	
tert-Butyl alcohol	CH$_3$	s	1.28	1.18	1.11	1.05	1.16	1.40	1.24
	OH	s			4.19	1.55	2.18		
tert-Butyl methyl ether	CCH$_3$	s	1.19	1.13	1.11	1.07	1.14	1.15	1.21
	OCH$_3$	s	3.22	3.13	3.08	3.04	3.13	3.20	3.22
BHT	ArH	s	6.98	6.96	6.87	7.05	6.97	6.92	
	OH	s	5.01		6.65	4.79	5.20		
	ArCH$_3$	s	2.27	2.22	2.18	2.24	2.22	2.21	
	ArC(CH$_3$)$_3$	s	1.43	1.41	1.36	1.38	1.39	1.40	
Chloroform	CH	s	7.26	8.02	8.32	6.15	7.58	7.90	
Cyclohexane	CH$_2$	s	1.43	1.43	1.40	1.40	1.44	1.45	
1,2-Dichloroethane	CH$_2$	s	3.73	3.87	3.90	2.90	3.81	3.78	
Dichloromethane	CH$_2$	s	5.30	5.63	5.76	4.27	5.44	5.49	
Diethyl ether	CH$_3$	t,7	1.21	1.11	1.09	1.11	1.12	1.18	1.17
	CH$_2$	q,7	3.48	3.41	3.38	3.26	3.42	3.49	3.56
Diglyme	CH$_2$	m	3.65	3.56	3.51	3.46	3.53	3.61	3.67
	CH$_2$	m	3.57	3.47	3.38	3.34	3.45	3.58	3.61
	OCH$_3$	s	3.39	3.28	3.24	3.11	3.29	3.35	3.37
1,2-Dimethoxyethane	CH$_3$	s	3.40	3.28	3.24	3.12	3.28	3.35	3.37
	CH$_2$	s	3.55	3.46	3.43	3.33	3.45	3.52	3.60
Dimethylacetamide	CH$_3$CO	s	2.09	1.97	1.96	1.60	1.97	2.07	2.08
	NCH$_3$	s	3.02	3.00	2.94	2.57	2.96	3.31	3.06

（续上表）

Solvent	proton	mult	CDCl$_3$	(CD$_3$)$_2$CO	(CD$_3$)$_2$SO	C$_6$D$_6$	CD$_3$CN	CD$_3$OD	D$_2$O
	NCH$_3$	s	2.94	2.83	2.78	2.05	2.83	2.92	2.90
Dimethylformamide	CH	s	8.02	7.96	7.95	7.63	7.92	7.97	7.92
	CH$_3$	s	2.96	2.94	2.89	2.36	2.89	2.99	3.01
	CH$_3$	s	2.88	2.78	2.73	1.86	2.77	2.86	2.85
Dimethyl sulfoxide	CH$_3$	s	2.62	2.52	2.54	1.68	2.50	2.65	2.71
Dioxane	CH$_2$	s	3.71	3.59	3.57	3.35	3.60	3.66	3.75
Ethanol	CH$_3$	t,7	1.25	1.12	1.06	0.96	1.12	1.19	1.17
	CH$_2$	q,7	3.72	3.57	3.44	3.34	3.54	3.60	3.65
	OH	s	1.32	3.39	4.63		2.47		
Ethyl acetate	CH$_3$CO	s	2.05	1.97	1.99	1.65	1.97	2.01	2.07
	CH$_2$CH$_3$	q,7	4.12	4.05	4.03	3.89	4.06	4.09	4.14
	CH$_2$CH$_3$	t,7	1.26	1.20	1.17	0.92	1.20	1.24	1.24
Ethyl methyl ketone	CH$_3$CO	s	2.14	2.07	2.07	1.58	2.06	2.12	2.19
	CH$_2$CH$_3$	q,7	2.46	2.45	2.43	1.81	2.43	2.50	3.18
	CH$_2$CH$_3$	t,7	1.06	0.96	0.91	0.85	0.96	1.01	1.26
Ethylene glycol	CH	s	3.76	3.28	3.34	3.41	3.51	3.59	3.65
"Grease"	CH$_3$	m	0.86	0.87		0.92	0.86	0.88	
	CH$_2$	br s	1.26	1.29		1.36	1.27	1.29	
n-Hexane	CH$_3$	t	0.88	0.88	0.86	0.89	0.89	0.90	
	CH$_2$	m	1.26	1.28	1.25	1.24	1.28	1.29	
HMPA	CH$_3$	d,9.5	2.65	2.59	2.53	2.40	2.57	2.64	2.61
Methanol	CH$_3$	s	3.49	3.31	3.16	3.07	3.28	3.34	3.34
	OH	s	1.09	3.12	4.01		2.16		
Nitromethane	CH$_3$	s	4.33	4.43	4.42	2.94	4.31	4.34	4.40
n-Pentane	CH$_3$	t,7	0.88	0.88	0.86	0.87	0.89	0.90	
	CH$_2$	m	1.27	1.27	1.27	1.23	1.29	1.29	
2-Propanol	CH$_3$	d,6	1.22	1.10	1.04	0.95	1.09	1.50	1.17
	CH	sep,6	4.04	3.90	3.78	3.67	3.87	3.92	4.02
Pyridine	CH (2)	m	8.62	8.58	8.58	8.53	8.57	8.53	8.52
	CH (3)	m	7.29	7.35	7.39	6.66	7.33	7.44	7.45
	CH (4)	m	7.68	7.76	7.79	6.98	7.73	7.85	7.87
Silicone grease	CH$_3$	s	0.07	0.13		0.29	0.08	0.10	

（续上表）

Solvent	proton	mult	CDCl₃	(CD₃)₂CO	(CD₃)₂SO	C₆D₆	CD₃CN	CD₃OD	D₂O
Tetrahydrofuran	CH₂	m	1.85	1.79	1.76	1.40	1.80	1.87	1.88
	CH₂O	m	3.76	3.63	3.60	3.57	3.64	3.71	3.74
Toluene	CH₃	s	2.36	2.32	2.30	2.11	2.33	2.32	
	CH (o/p)	m	7.17	7.1 −7.2	7.18	7.02	7.1	−7.3	7.16
	CH (m)	m	7.25	7.1 −7.2	7.25	7.13	7.1	−7.3	7.16
Triethylamine	CH₃	t,7	1.03	0.96	0.93	0.96	0.96	1.05	0.99
	CH₂	q,7	2.53	2.45	2.43	2.40	2.45	2.58	2.57

^{13}C-NMR Data

Solvent		CDCl₃	(CD₃)₂CO	(CD₃)₂SO	C₆D₆	CD₃CN	CD₃OD	D₂O
Solvent signals		77.16 ± 0.06	29.84 ± 0.01	39.52 ± 0.06	128.06 ± 0.02	1.32 ± 0.02	49.00 ± 0.01	
			206.26 ± 0.13		118.26 ± 0.02			
Acetic acid	CO	175.99	172.31	171.93	175.82	173.21	175.11	177.21
	CH₃	20.81	20.51	20.95	20.37	20.73	20.56	21.03
Acetone	CO	207.07	205.87	206.31	204.43	207.43	209.67	215.94
	CH₃	30.92	30.60	30.56	30.14	30.91	30.67	30.89
Acetonitrile	CN	116.43	117.60	117.91	116.02	118.26	118.06	119.68
	CH₃	1.89	1.12	1.03	0.20	1.79	0.85	1.47
Benzene	CH	128.37	129.15	128.30	128.62	129.32	129.34	
tert-Butyl alcohol	C	69.15	68.13	66.88	68.19	68.74	69.40	70.36
	CH₃	31.25	30.72	30.38	30.47	30.68	30.91	30.29
tert-Butyl methyl ether	OCH₃	49.45	49.35	48.70	49.19	49.52	49.66	49.37
	C	72.87	72.81	72.04	72.40	73.17	74.32	75.62
	C CH₃	26.99	27.24	26.79	27.09	27.28	27.22	26.60
BHT	C (1)	151.55	152.51	151.47	152.05	152.42	152.85	
	C (2)	135.87	138.19	139.12	136.08	138.13	139.09	
	CH (3)	125.55	129.05	127.97	128.52	129.61	129.49	
	C (4)	128.27	126.03	124.85	125.83	126.38	126.11	
	CH₃ Ar	21.20	21.31	20.97	21.40	21.23	21.38	
	CH₃ C	30.33	31.61	31.25	31.34	31.50	31.15	

（续上表）

Solvent		CDCl$_3$	(CD$_3$)$_2$CO	(CD$_3$)$_2$SO	C$_6$D$_6$	CD$_3$CN	CD$_3$OD	D$_2$O
	C	34.25	35.00	34.33	34.35	35.05	35.36	
Chloroform	CH	77.36	79.19	79.16	77.79	79.17	79.44	
Cyclohexane	CH$_2$	26.94	27.51	26.33	27.23	27.63	27.96	
1,2-Dichloroethane	CH$_2$	43.50	45.25	45.02	43.59	45.54	45.11	
Dichloromethane	CH$_2$	53.52	54.95	54.84	53.46	55.32	54.78	
Diethyl ether	CH$_3$	15.20	15.78	15.12	15.46	15.63	15.46	14.77
	CH$_2$	65.91	66.12	62.05	65.94	66.32	66.88	66.42
Diglyme	CH$_3$	59.01	58.77	57.98	58.66	58.90	59.06	58.67
	CH$_2$	70.51	71.03	69.54	70.87	70.99	71.33	70.05
	CH$_2$	71.90	72.63	71.25	72.35	72.63	72.92	71.63
1,2-Dimethoxyethane	CH$_3$	59.08	58.45	58.01	58.68	58.89	59.06	58.67
	CH$_2$	71.84	72.47	17.07	72.21	72.47	72.72	71.49
Dimethylacetamide	CH$_3$	21.53	21.51	21.29	21.16	21.76	21.32	21.09
	CO	171.07	170.61	169.54	169.95	171.31	173.32	174.57
	NCH$_3$	35.28	34.89	37.38	34.67	35.17	35.50	35.03
	NCH$_3$	38.13	37.92	34.42	37.03	38.26	38.43	38.76
Dimethylformamide	CH	162.62	162.79	162.29	162.13	163.31	164.73	165.53
	CH$_3$	36.50	36.15	35.73	35.25	36.57	36.89	37.54
	CH$_3$	31.45	31.03	30.73	30.72	31.32	31.61	32.03
Dimethyl sulfoxide	CH$_3$	40.76	41.23	40.45	40.03	41.31	40.45	39.39
Dioxane	CH$_2$	67.14	67.60	66.36	67.16	67.72	68.11	67.19
Ethanol	CH$_3$	18.41	18.89	18.51	18.72	18.80	18.40	17.47
	CH$_2$	58.28	57.72	56.07	57.86	57.96	58.26	58.05
Ethyl acetate	CH$_3$CO	21.04	20.83	20.68	20.56	21.16	20.88	21.15
	CO	171.36	170.96	170.31	170.44	171.68	172.89	175.26
	CH$_2$	60.49	60.56	59.74	60.21	60.98	61.50	62.32
	CH$_3$	14.19	14.50	14.40	14.19	14.54	14.49	13.92
Ethyl methyl ketone	CH$_3$CO	29.49	29.30	29.26	28.56	29.60	29.39	29.49
	CO	209.56	208.30	208.72	206.55	209.88	212.16	218.43
	CH$_2$CH$_3$	36.89	36.75	35.83	36.36	37.09	37.34	37.27
	CH$_2$CH$_3$	7.86	8.03	7.61	7.91	8.14	8.09	7.87
Ethylene glycol	CH$_2$	63.79	64.26	62.76	64.34	64.22	64.30	63.17

（续上表）

Solvent		CDCl$_3$	(CD$_3$)$_2$CO	(CD$_3$)$_2$SO	C$_6$D$_6$	CD$_3$CN	CD$_3$OD	D$_2$O
"Grease"	CH$_2$	29.76	30.73	29.20	30.21	30.86	31.29	
n-Hexane	CH$_3$	14.14	14.34	13.88	14.32	14.43	14.45	
	CH$_2$(2)	22.70	23.28	22.05	23.04	23.40	23.68	
	CH$_2$(3)	31.64	32.30	30.95	31.96	32.36	32.73	
HMPA	CH$_3$	36.87	37.04	36.42	36.88	37.10	37.00	36.46
Methanol	CH$_3$	50.41	49.77	48.59	49.97	49.90	49.86	49.50
Nitromethane	CH$_3$	62.50	63.21	63.28	61.16	63.66	63.08	63.22
n-Pentane	CH$_3$	14.08	14.29	13.28	14.25	14.37	14.39	
	CH$_2$(2)	22.38	22.98	21.70	22.72	23.08	23.38	
	CH$_2$(3)	34.16	34.83	33.48	34.45	34.89	35.30	
2-Propanol	CH$_3$	25.14	25.67	25.43	25.18	25.55	25.27	24.38
	CH	64.50	63.85	64.92	64.23	64.30	64.71	64.88
Pyridine	CH (2)	149.90	150.67	149.58	150.27	150.76	150.07	149.18
	CH (3)	123.75	124.57	123.84	123.58	127.76	125.53	125.12
	CH (4)	135.96	136.56	136.05	135.28	136.89	138.35	138.27
Silicone grease	CH$_3$	1.04	1.40		1.38		2.10	
Tetrahydrofuran	CH$_2$	25.62	26.15	25.14	25.72	26.27	26.48	25.67
	CH$_2$O	67.97	68.07	67.03	67.80	68.33	68.83	68.68
Toluene	CH$_3$	21.46	21.46	20.99	21.10	21.50	21.50	
	C (i)	137.89	138.48	137.35	137.91	138.90	138.85	
	CH (o)	129.07	129.76	128.88	129.33	129.94	129.91	
	CH (m)	128.26	129.03	128.18	128.56	129.23	129.20	
	CH (p)	125.33	126.12	125.29	125.68	126.28	126.29	
Triethylamine	CH$_3$	11.61	12.49	11.74	12.35	12.38	11.09	9.07
	CH$_2$	46.25	47.07	45.74	46.77	47.10	46.96	47.19

参考文献

［1］GOTTLIEB H E, KOTLYAR V, NUDELMAN A. NMR chemical shifts of common laboratory solvents as trace impurities［J］. The journal of organic chemistry, 1997, 62 (21):7512 – 7515.

附录 5　常见质子类型 ^{1}H-NMR 的化学位移

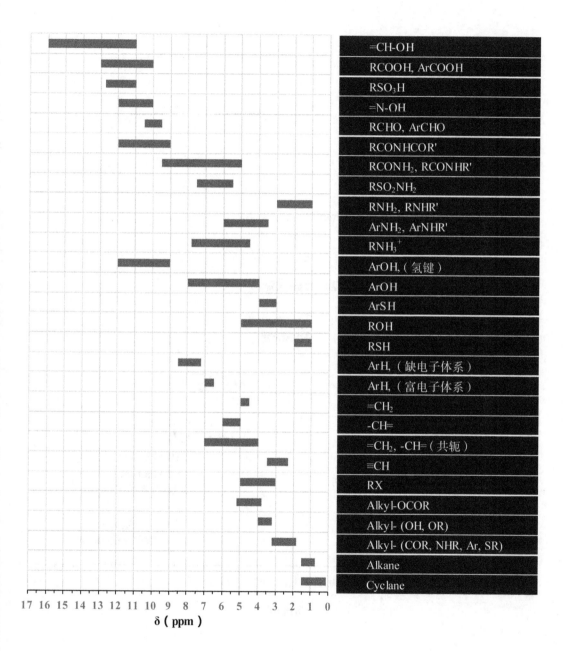

附录6 常见不同类型碳^{13}C-NMR 的化学位移

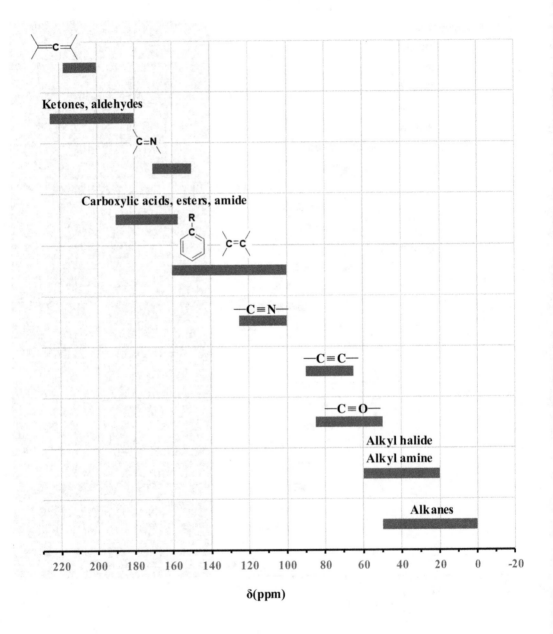

δ(ppm)

附录7　常见有机功能团的红外谱带参考图表

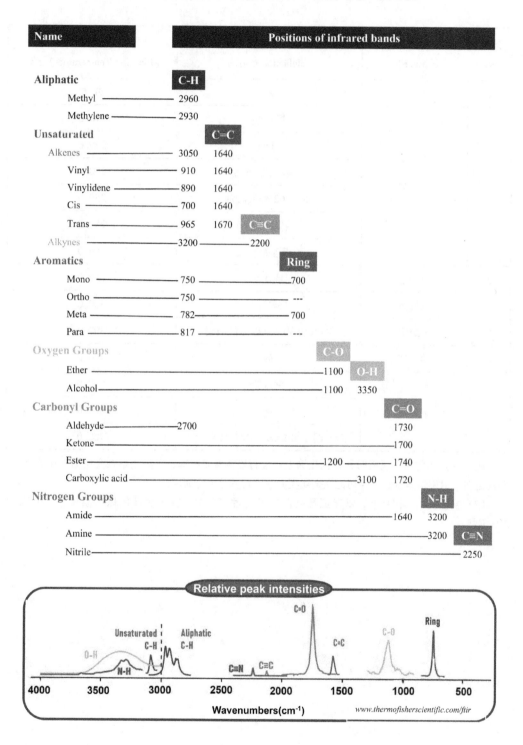

附录 8   常用加热浴种类

序号 （No.）	名称 （Name）	加热载体 （Calefaction Carrier）	极限温度 （Limiting Temperature）/℃
1	水 浴	水	98.0
2	油 浴	棉籽油	210.0
		甘油	220.0
		液状石蜡	220.0
		58～62号汽缸油	250.0
		甲基硅油	250.0
		苯基硅油	300.0
3	硫酸浴	H_2SO_4	250.0
4	空气浴	空气	300.0
5	石蜡浴	熔点为30～60℃的石蜡	300.0
6	砂 浴	砂	400.0
7	金属浴	铜或铅	500.0
		锡	600.0
		铝青铜（90% Cu、10% Al合金）	700.0

注：（1）在使用金属浴时，要预先涂上一层石墨在器皿底部，以防止熔融金属黏附在器皿上，尤其是在使用玻璃器皿时；要切记在金属凝固前应将其移出金属浴。

（2）初次使用的棉籽油，要保证最高温度不超过180℃，在多次使用以后温度才可升高到210℃。

附录9　常用冷却剂

一种盐和水或冰组成的冷却剂

序号 （No.）	盐 （Salt）	X/g	△t/℃	Y/g	冰盐点 （Cryohydric point）/℃
1	$CaCl_2$	250.0	23.0	42.2	−55.0
2	$CaCl_2 \cdot 6H_2O$	—	—	41.0	−9.0
3	$CaCl_2 \cdot 6H_2O$	—	—	82.0	−21.5
4	$CaCl_2 \cdot 6H_2O$	—	—	100.0	−29.0
5	$CaCl_2 \cdot 6H_2O$	—	—	125.0	−40.3
6	$CaCl_2 \cdot 6H_2O$	—	—	150.0	−49.0
7	$CaCl_2 \cdot 6H_2O$	—	—	500.0	−54.0
8	$CaCl_2 \cdot 6H_2O$	—	—	143.0	−55.0
9	$FeCl_2$	—	—	49.7	−55.0
10	$MgCl_2$	—	—	27.5	−33.6
11	NaCl	36.0	2.5	30.4	−21.2
12	$(NH_4)_2SO_4$	75.0	6.0	62.0	−19.0
13	$NaNO_3$	75.0	18.5	59.0	−18.5
14	NH_4NO_3	100.0	27.0	50.0	−17.0
15	NH_4Cl	30.0	18.0	25.0	−15.0
16	KCl	30.0	13.0	30.0	−11.0
17	$Na_2S_2O_3$	70.0	18.7	42.8	−11.0
18	$MgSO_4$	85.0	8.0	23.4	−3.9
19	KNO_3	16.0	10.0	13.0	−2.9
20	Na_2CO_3	40.0	9.0	6.3	−2.1
21	K_2SO_4	12.0	3.0	6.5	−1.6
22	CH_3COONa	51.1	15.4	—	—
23	KSCN	150.0	34.5	—	—
24	NH_4Cl	133.0	31.2	29.7	−15.8

（续上表）

序号 （No.）	盐 （Salt）	X/g	△t/℃	Y/g	冰盐点 （Cryohydric point）/℃
25	$(NH_4)_2CO_3$	30.0	12.0	—	
26	$Na_2SO_4 \cdot 10\,H_2O$	20.0	7.0	—	
27	NH_4SCN	133.0	31.0	—	
28	$Pb(NO_3)_2$	—	—	54.3	-2.7
29	$ZnSO_4$	—	—	37.4	-6.6
30	$ZnCl_2$	—	—	108.3	-62.0
31	K_2CO_3	—	—	65.3	-36.5
32	$BaCl_2$	—	—	40.8	-7.8
33	$MnSO_4$	—	—	90.5	-10.5

注：X（g）盐和100 g水在10～15 ℃时混合，温度降低△t（℃）。Y（g）盐和100 g冰混合，温度将降到冰盐点。

附录 10　常用干燥剂

序号 (No.)	名称 (Name)	分子式 (Molecular Formula)	吸水能力 (Moisture Absorption Capacity)	干燥速度 (Drying Speed)	酸碱性 (Acidity and Alkaline)	再生方式 (Regenerative Way)
1	硫酸钙	$CaSO_4$	小	快	中性	在 163 ℃（脱水温度）下脱水再生
2	氧化钡	BaO	—	慢	碱性	不能再生
3	五氧化二磷	P_2O_5	大	快	酸性	不能再生
4	氯化钙（熔融过的）	$CaCl_2$	大	快	含碱性杂质	200 ℃下烘干再生
5	高氯酸镁	$Mg(ClO_4)_2$	大	快	中性	烘干再生（251 ℃分解）
6	三水合高氯酸镁	$Mg(ClO_4)_2 \cdot 3H_2O$	—	快	中性	烘干再生（251 ℃分解）
7	氢氧化钾（熔融过的）	KOH	大	较快	碱性	不能再生
8	活性氧化铝	Al_2O_3	大	快	中性	在 110～300 ℃下烘干再生
9	浓硫酸	H_2SO_4	大	快	酸性	蒸发浓缩再生
10	硅胶	SiO_2	大	快	酸性	120 ℃下烘干再生
11	氢氧化钠（熔融过的）	$NaOH$	大	较快	碱性	不能再生
12	氧化钙	CaO	—	慢	碱性	不能再生
13	硫酸铜	$CuSO_4$	大	—	微酸性	150 ℃下烘干再生
14	硫酸镁	$MgSO_4$	大	较快	中性、有的微酸性	200 ℃下烘干再生
15	硫酸钠	Na_2SO_4	大	慢	中性	烘干再生
16	碳酸钾	K_2CO_3	中	较慢	碱性	100 ℃下烘干再生
17	金属钠	Na	—	—	—	不能再生
18	分子筛	结晶的铝硅酸盐	大	较快	酸性	烘干，温度随型号而异

注：使用高氯酸盐时务必小心，碳、硫、磷及一切有机物都不能与之接触，否则会发生猛烈爆炸，造成危险。

附录11　干燥适用条件

序号 （No.）	名称 （Name）	适用物质 （Applicable Substance）	不适用物质 （Inapplicable Substance）	备注 （Remark）
1	碱石灰 氧化钡、氧化钙	中性和碱性气体，胺类，醇类，醚类	醛类，酮类，酸性物质	特别适用于干燥气体，与水作用生成 $Ba(OH)_2$、$Ca(OH)_2$
2	硫酸钙	普遍适用	—	常先用 H_2SO_4 钠作预干燥剂
3	氢氧化钠、氢氧化钾	氨，胺类，醚类，烃类（干燥器），肼类，碱类	醛类，酮类，酸性物质	容易潮解，一般用于预干燥
4	碳酸钾	胺类，醇类，丙酮，一般的生物碱类，酯类，腈类，肼类，卤素衍生物	酸类，酚类及其他酸性物质	容易潮解
5	氯化钙	烷烃类，链烯烃类，醚类，酯类，卤代烃类，腈类，丙酮，醛类，硝基化合物类，中性气体，氯化氢，二氧化碳	醇类，氨，胺类，酸类，酸性物质，某些醛，酮类与酯类	一种价格便宜的干燥剂，可与许多含氮、含氧的化合物生成溶剂化物、络合物或发生反应；一般含有 CaO 等碱性杂质
6	五氧化二磷	大多数中性和酸性气体，乙炔，二硫化碳，烃类，各种卤代烃，酸溶液，酸与酸酐，腈类	碱性物质，醇类，酮类，醚类，易发生聚合的物质，氯化氢，氟化氢，氨气	使用其干燥气体时必须与载体或填料（石棉绒、玻璃棉、浮石等）混合；一般先用其他干燥剂预干燥；本品易潮解，与水作用生成偏磷酸、磷酸等
7	浓硫酸	大多数中性与酸性气体（干燥器、洗气瓶），各种饱和烃，卤代烃，芳烃	不饱和的有机化合物，醇类，酮类，酚类，碱性物质，硫化氢（H_2S），碘化氢（HI），氨气（NH_3）	不适宜升温干燥和真空干燥
8	金属钠	醚类，饱和烃类，叔胺类，芳烃类	氯代烃类（会发生爆炸危险），醇类，伯、仲胺类及其他易和金属钠起作用的物质	一般先用其他干燥剂预干燥，与水作用生成 NaOH 与 H_2
9	硫酸钠、硫酸镁	普遍适用，特别适用于酯类，酮类及一些敏感物溶液	—	一种价格便宜的干燥剂；（Na_2SO_4）常作预干燥剂
10	硅胶	置于干燥器中使用	氟化氢	加热干燥后可重复使用
11	分子筛	温度 100 ℃ 以下的大多数流动气体；有机溶剂（干燥器）	不饱和烃	一般先用其他干燥剂预干燥，特别适用于低分压的干燥

（续上表）

序号 （No.）	名称 （Name）	适用物质 （Applicable Substance）	不适用物质 （Inapplicable Substance）	备注 （Remark）
12	氢化钙	烃类，醚类，酯类，C_4 及 C_4 以上的醇类	醛类，含有活泼羰基的化合物	作用比 $LiAlH_4$ 漫，但效率相近，且较安全，是最好的脱水剂之一，与水作用生成 $Ca(OH)_2$ 与 H_2
13	四氢铝锂	烃类，芳基卤化物，醚类	含有酸性 H，卤素，羰基及硝基等的化合物	使用时要小心。过剩的可以慢慢加乙酸乙酯将其破坏；与水作用生成 $LiOH$、$Al(OH)_3$ 与 H_2

附录12　元素周期表

1 Group IA	2 IIA												13 IIIB IIIA	14 IVB IVA	15 VB VA	16 VIB VIA	17 VIIB VIIA	18 VIIIA	Shell
1 H +1 -1 1.007941 1																		2 He 4.002602 2	K
3 Li +1 6.941 2-1	4 Be +2 9.012182 2-2				Key to Chart Atomic Number →50 +2 +4 ← Oxidation States Symbol →Sn 2001 Atomic Weight →118.710 -18-18-4 ← Electron Configuration								5 B +3 10.811 2-3	6 C +2 +4 -4 12.0107 2-4	7 N +1 +2 +3 +4 +5 -3 14.0067 2-5	8 O -2 15.9994 2-6	9 F -1 18.9984032 2-7	10 Ne 20.1797 2-8	K-L
11 Na +1 22.989770 2-8-1	12 Mg +2 24.3050 2-8-2	3 IIIA IIIB	4 IVA IVB	5 VA VB	6 VIA VIB	7 VIIA VIIB	8	9 VIIIA VIII	10	11 IB IB	12 IIB IIB	13 Al +3 26.981538 2-8-3	14 Si +2 +4 -4 28.0855 2-8-4	15 P +3 +5 -3 30.973761 2-8-5	16 S +4 +6 -2 32.065 2-8-6	17 Cl +1 +5 +7 -1 35.453 2-8-7	18 Ar 39.948 2-8-8	K-L-M
19 K +1 39.0983 -8-8-1	20 Ca +2 40.078 -8-8-2	21 Sc +3 44.955910 -8-9-2	22 Ti +2 +3 +4 47.867 -8-10-2	23 V +2 +3 +4 +5 50.9415 -8-11-2	24 Cr +2 +3 +6 51.9961 -8-13-1	25 Mn +2 +3 +4 +6 +7 54.938049 -8-13-2	26 Fe +2 +3 55.845 -8-14-2	27 Co +2 +3 58.933200 -8-15-2	28 Ni +2 +3 58.6934 -8-16-2	29 Cu +1 +2 63.546 -8-18-1	30 Zn +2 65.409 -8-18-2	31 Ga +3 69.723 -8-18-3	32 Ge +2 +4 72.64 -8-18-4	33 As +3 +5 -3 74.92160 -8-18-5	34 Se +4 +6 -2 78.96 -8-18-6	35 Br +1 +5 -1 79.904 -8-18-7	36 Kr 83.798 -8-18-8	-L-M-N
37 Rb +1 85.4678 -18-8-1	38 Sr +2 87.62 -18-8-2	39 Y +3 88.90585 -18-9-2	40 Zr +4 91.224 -18-10-2	41 Nb +3 +5 92.90638 -18-12-1	42 Mo +6 95.94 -18-13-1	43 Tc +4 +6 +7 (98) -18-13-2	44 Ru +3 101.07 -18-15-1	45 Rh +3 102.90550 -18-16-1	46 Pd +2 +4 106.42 -18-18-0	47 Ag +1 107.8682 -18-18-1	48 Cd +2 112.411 -18-18-2	49 In +3 114.818 -18-18-3	50 Sn +2 +4 118.710 -18-18-4	51 Sb +3 +5 -3 121.760 -18-18-5	52 Te +4 +6 -2 127.60 -18-18-6	53 I +1 +5 +7 -1 126.90447 -18-18-7	54 Xe 0 131.293 -18-18-8	-M-N-O
55 Cs +1 132.90545 -18-8-1	56 Ba +2 137.327 -18-8-2	57* La +3 138.9055 -18-9-2	72 Hf +4 178.49 -32-10-2	73 Ta +5 180.9479 -32-11-2	74 W +6 183.84 -32-12-2	75 Re +4 +6 +7 186.207 -32-13-2	76 Os +3 +4 190.23 -32-14-2	77 Ir +3 +4 192.217 -32-15-2	78 Pt +2 +4 195.078 -32-17-1	79 Au +1 +3 196.96655 -32-18-1	80 Hg +1 +2 200.59 -32-18-2	81 Tl +1 +3 204.3833 -32-18-3	82 Pb +2 +4 207.2 -32-18-4	83 Bi +3 +5 208.98038 -32-18-5	84 Po +2 +4 (209) -32-18-6	85 At -1 (210) -32-18-7	86 Rn 0 (222) -32-18-8	-N-O-P
87 Fr +1 (223) -18-8-1	88 Ra +2 (226) -18-8-2	89** Ac +3 (227) -18-9-2	104 Rf +4 (261) -32-10-2	105 Db (262) -32-11-2	106 Sg (266) -32-12-2	107 Bh (264) -32-13-2	108 Hs (277) -32-14-2	109 Mt (268) -32-15-2	110 Ds (271) -32-16-2	111 Rg (272)	112 Uub (285)		114 Uuq (289)			116 Uuh (289)		-O-P-Q

* Lanthanides	58 Ce +3 +4 140.116 -19-9-2	59 Pr +3 140.90765 -21-8-2	60 Nd +3 144.24 -22-8-2	61 Pm +3 (145) -23-8-2	62 Sm +2 +3 150.36 -24-8-2	63 Eu +2 +3 151.964 -25-8-2	64 Gd +3 157.25 -25-9-2	65 Tb +3 158.92534 -27-8-2	66 Dy +3 162.500 -28-8-2	67 Ho +3 164.93032 -29-8-2	68 Er +3 167.259 -30-8-2	69 Tm +3 168.93421 -31-8-2	70 Yb +2 +3 173.04 -32-8-2	71 Lu +3 174.967 -32-9-2		-N-O-P
** Actinides	90 Th +4 232.0381 -18-10-2	91 Pa +4 +5 231.03588 -20-9-2	92 U +3 +4 +5 +6 238.02891 -21-9-2	93 Np +3 +4 +5 +6 (237) -22-9-2	94 Pu +3 +4 +5 +6 (244) -24-8-2	95 Am +3 +4 +5 +6 (243) -25-8-2	96 Cm +3 (247) -25-9-2	97 Bk +3 +4 (247) -27-8-2	98 Cf +3 (251) -28-8-2	99 Es +3 (252) -29-8-2	100 Fm +3 (257) -30-8-2	101 Md +2 +3 (258) -31-8-2	102 No +2 +3 (259) -32-8-2	103 Lr +3 (262) -32-8-3		-O-P-Q

New Notation ——— ← 13 IIIB / IIIA
Previous IUPAC Form ——— 14 IVB / IVA 15 VB / VA 16 VIB / VIA 17 VIIB / VIIA 18 VIIIA
CAS Version ———

The new IUPAC format numbers the groups from 1 to 18. The previous IUPAC numbering system and the system used by Chemical Abstracts Service (CAS) are also shown. For radioactive elements that do not occur in nature, the mass number of the most stable isotope is given in parentheses. Elements 112, 114, and 116 have been reported but not confirmed.

☐ Metallic solids　　☐ Non-metallic solids

☐ Liquids　　☐ Gases

附录 13　药物化学实验仪器清单

序号	品　名	数量	序号	品名	数量
1	三颈烧瓶，250mL	1	26	温度计套24#	1
2	三颈烧瓶，100mL	1	27	搅拌子（小、中）	2
3	茄形瓶/圆底烧瓶，500mL	1	28	量筒，10mL	1
4	圆底烧瓶，250mL	1	29	量筒，100mL	1
5	圆底烧瓶，100mL	2	30	点样毛细管	1
6	抽滤瓶，250mL	1	31	剪刀	1
7	布氏漏斗	1	32	镊子	1
8	抽滤套垫	1	33	牛角匙	1
9	长玻璃漏斗	1	34	不锈钢匙	1
10	短玻璃漏斗	1	35	刮铲	1
11	锥形瓶，50mL	1	36	长玻璃棒	1
12	锥形瓶，100mL	1	37	短玻璃棒	1
13	锥形瓶，100mL	1	38	酒精温度计	2
14	锥形瓶，250mL	1	39	吸磁搅拌棒	1
15	展缸	1	40	球形冷凝管	1
16	烧杯，100mL	2	41	黑色烧瓶垫	2
17	烧杯，250mL	1			
18	磁蒸发皿	1			
19	洗耳球	1			
20	表面皿	1			
21	培养皿	2			
22	pH试纸	1			
23	磁六孔板	1			
24	防溅球	2			
25	空心塞24#	4			